D1807688

A Meaningful Year

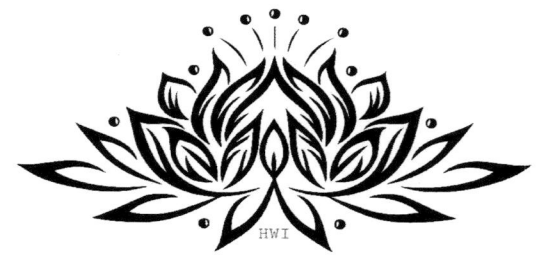

Copyright© Jo Wren 2018

All rights reserved.

ISBN: 9781797946849

All Rights Reserved. No part of this publication may be reproduced, stored in a retrieval system, or transmitted in any form, or by any means, electronic, mechanical, photocopying, recording or otherwise without the prior permission in writing of the copyright holders, nor be otherwise circulated in any form or binding or cover other than in which it is published and without a similar condition being imposed on the subsequent publisher.

A Meaningful Year

An Occupational Therapy based approach to Health and Well-Being

Jo Wren

Contents

This is a lovely warming crumble for those cold autumn days and one of my favourite recipes. If you haven't baked before, this is a good one to start with. I remember making apple crumble at school and proudly carrying it home.

These pretty little biscuits are easy to make and taste great. The lemon flavour works well with the sweetness of the icing. They are crumbly like shortbread and go well with a cup of tea.

This is an easy savoury scone recipe. It was the first savoury scone recipe I tried and smells amazing whilst it's cooking. This recipe makes one round that can be cut into approximately 8 individual scones.

This idea is great if you want easy access to fresh herbs to use in your kitchen. It also means that you can grow even if you have limited or no outdoor space, all you need is a windowsill.

This is also a great idea for engaging with nature if you have limited outdoor space. If you have no outdoor space choose indoor plants and see the "Connect with nature" suggestion box for more ideas for indoor instant gardens. It can be planted with seeds to reduce the cost, but if you want an instant garden, use small plants.

Growing your own vegetables can reduce the cost of grocery bills, support a healthy diet and be rewarding. Waiting times for allotments can be long and it can be hard to manage one if you have other time commitments, so why not start your own in pots. It can be taken with you if you move too.

By noticing what is around us, we become mindful of our surroundings. Mindful photography can help us to focus, concentrate, express ourselves creatively and be curious. I have used mindful photography as a therapeutic tool when working with people with depression and anxiety as it helps to focus the mind on the environment rather than on anxious or negative thoughts.

Still life photography can be used as a mindful meditation by looking. It is taking the time to really explore what you are seeing.

This project involves going to your favourite place with your phone or camera and capturing the beauty of it to make images that remind you of that place at other, perhaps more stressful times. I use them as screen savers at work.

This is a warming thick soup, full of flavour. It's a versatile recipe for any time of the year, just use whatever vegetables are seasonal.

This is an easy colourful salad with sweet and savoury flavours. The edible flowers add interest and colour to the dish as well as providing subtle flavours that you can be mindful when tasting.

This chutney goes really well with cheese and has Christmassy flavours as it uses ginger and nutmeg, but the recipe can be easily adapted for other times of the year.

This project captures the forms of nature in detail and can be adapted to match your favourite colours. It can also be made into a keychain by attaching it to the hook from a pound token.

It's lovely to spend time outside on a fair weather day, but by doing this project you'll also have a lovely textile piece to take home with you.

This project incorporates a walk on a beach, mindfully looking for "treasures" to take home and create something beautiful to remind you of the day.

This project involves using the beauty of natural objects to make art and is a great activity to do with your children.

The mandala (translated as "circle") is a Tibetan Buddhist visual aid for concentration and meditation. You don't need to follow the Buddhist faith to make a mandala, but ideas from other faiths and cultures can add to our toolbox of occupations that we find therapeutic.

This project is fun to do at Easter, but can be done any time of the year to make unique and colourful ornaments. The use of natural dyes is creative and can give unusual and unpredictable results.

The following project involves using writing as a medium to help us to connect with nature and be more mindful but there are also suggestions to help you make it more social and creative.

This project involves writing about an experience in a short poem. At first I found it restricting and a bit frustrating, but with some practice I think it teaches us to be succinct and consider each word carefully.

One of the ways of connecting more with nature that I've found useful is to take my journal out when I go for a walk somewhere beautiful in nature and take a moment to describe where I am in a short piece of writing that uses as many of the senses as possible. By doing this I find that I am naturally being more mindful as I am focussed on the present moment and not my thoughts.

Acknowledgements

My deepest gratitude goes to all the clients it's been my absolute privilege to work with so far in my career.

The Health and Well-being Initiative, our team occupational therapy adventure has re-energised my career, so a heartfelt thank you goes to my colleagues Sian Kirkland Harris, Julie Rowbottom, Karen Thakuria, and everyone who supported us to start out. To find out more about the initiative visit https://thehealthandwell-be-inginitiative.wordpress.com

Many thanks as well to the following people for feedback and encouragement to make the final resource everything I wanted it to be: Amanda Jackson, Zoe Corbridge, Jane Cronin-Davis, Lou Bellingham, Donna Stone, Karen Thakuria, Sian Kirkland-Harris and Julie Rowbottom.

Jo Wren *BSc(Hons), PGCert, MSc, RCOT, RCOTSS-Independent Practice, HCPC.*

Introduction

It can be difficult to find time to look after ourselves. However, if we use an analogy and think of ourselves as a leaky bucket, with all the things we need to do as the holes in the bucket and the water as our mental and physical health and well-being and resilience, we need to keep filling the bucket or replenishing ourselves to be able to do all the things that we need to do in our lives. Our physical and mental health is what enables us to do the things we need to do, and well-being (our feelings of being healthy and happy) is what helps us to live a good quality of life. This resource was created by drawing together evidence and guidance from the occupational therapy literature, from the recovery literature in mental health, from my experience of my own mental health recovery journey, from working with clients guiding them on their journey, and from working with highly skilled colleagues. It draws together a model of how meaningful activity or *occupation* can promote health and well-being and how this can be applied to everyday life in practical ways through a series of projects and ideas to take our practice further into routines that make up our lifestyle. Although much of the research is based on mental health and well-being, mental and physical health and well-being are not separate, so improvement in mental health will have a positive impact on physical health as well

and the World Health Organisations definition of health as "*a state of complete physical, mental and social well-being not merely the absence of disease or infirmity*" (WHO 2019) illustrates this holistic view.

My aim is to make theory and ideas accessible to everyone by focussing on the application of the art and science of occupational therapy and introducing a number of projects where you can have a go and find out for yourself the therapeutic value of activities that are meaningful to you personally. If you would like to read further about occupational therapy, visit the Royal College of Occupational Therapists website at https://www.rcot.co.uk

1. Defining occupation

Occupational therapy is a health profession underpinned by occupational science and allied to medicine that can be found in many fields of clinical practice around the world, for example; paediatrics, learning difficulties, mental health, neurology, orthotics, equipment and adaptations and increasingly many other non-traditional settings such as the impact of being displaced in homelessness and refugeeism. Unique to the profession is the concept of *occupation* and its relationship to health and well-being. Occupation in this context is not used to describe just the worker role that a person has, but your *life's work*, or what we do to be who we are and become what we need to be. Our beliefs about occupation form the basis of our thinking about causes of ill health and our approach to assessment and treatment in health and well-being. Anne Wilcox, an occupational therapist, provides a useful definition of the term occupation below when she writes;

"People have an intrinsic drive to be active that is expressed through the occupations that form the fabric of their daily lives. Occupation is the term used to describe all the things that people do in everyday life, including caring for themselves and others, working, learning, playing, creating and interacting with other people. Occupation is central to the existence of individuals, groups and communities. It is the mechanism by which people maintain themselves in the world and realise their potential"
(Wilcox 1998)

The Royal College of Occupational Therapists (formally the College of Occupational Therapists) below describes some of the many reasons that occupational therapists believe that people engage in occupations and the possible consequences of being unable to perform occupations or *occupational deprivation* due to for example,

homelessness or displacement, illness, geographical isolation, incarceration etc

"Through what they do, people develop skills, exercise, and test their capacities, interact with others, adapt to circumstances, meet basic vital needs, express who they are and strive towards their goals. If a person is deprived of activity, or has access to a limited range of occupations, physical and psychological health will suffer.....Maintaining an acceptable and personally satisfying routine of activities that have meaning and value for the individual gives a structure to time and creates a sense of purpose and direction in life"
(COT Recovering Ordinary Lives 2006)

Reilly (1962) defined the occupational therapy hypothesis as; "*That man, through the use of his hands as they are energised by mind and will, can influence the state of his own health*". Here she suggests that health can be maintained by a continued interaction with the environment through doing. Reilly also suggests that this occurs through the mechanism of central nervous system adaption, and that by using acquired skills and creativity man can "*deploy his thinking, feelings and purpose to make himself at home in the world and make the world his home*". Here occupation is defined in terms of an adaptive response that facilitates the development of skills which then lead to health and well-being due to a fit between the person and the environment. A model of practice is a summary of a theory, and many models of practice in occupational therapy consider the person, interacting with the environment by doing the occupation, making practice both holistic and person centred.

A study by Clark et al (1997) provides strong evidence for a link between engagement in meaningful occupation and positive health experiences. In the Well Elderly study, three hundred and sixty one independent living, culturally diverse volunteers aged sixty or over were randomised into three groups. The intervention group (n=122) completed an occupational intervention that focused on health through occupation and the importance of meaningful activity in their lives. A social activity group (n=120) were included to control for therapist contact effects and took part in social activities such as dancing and walks. A non-intervention control group (n=119) received no therapist contact. After a nine month period, results showed that the intervention group scored significantly higher on fifteen out of twenty self reported outcome measures of functional status, life satisfaction, medical outcomes, social functioning and general mental health. Clark suggests that the positive health effects were due to individualised treatment plans that focused on occupations that were meaningful to participants.

In terms of our own personal experience, we may have experienced occupational deprivation and the effects of this, but if we have not, we have all probably experienced temporary *occupational disruption* as a result of being unwell for a time. If we think about having influenza and spending time in bed out of our normal routine, not seeing the people we usually socialise, work or study with, not feeling able to do the things that make us feel like we have accomplished something and reached our goals that day, the effect although temporary can give us an insight into why what we do is important to us. A period of physical ill health can also affect our mental health and make us feel low in mood, demonstrating the holistic nature of physical and mental health being fundamentally linked.

In my career as an occupational therapist, I have worked with clients of all ages in physical health, mental health and learning difficulty settings who were referred to me because they were having difficulty doing what they need to do in their everyday lives for a variety of reasons. One of the main aims of occupational therapy is to help people to become or remain as independent as possible in the areas that they choose to do so.

Part of my role as an occupational therapist involves *activity analysis* to find out what is stopping a person from engaging in the occupations that they usually do. Below I've given an example of an activity analysis, as seen by an occupational therapist, of making a cup of tea to illustrate the *occupational performance components* involved. Occupational performance components are the skills, knowledge and experience we utilise to perform an occupation and fall into the categories of; sensori-motor, motor, cognitive, psychological and social.

Steps in making a cup of tea:

1. Recognise that you are thirsty (receiving and interpreting correctly signals from the body).

2. Know that you need to drink to stop being thirsty (problem solving).

3. Decide to make yourself a drink now (decision making, motivation, initiation of activity, correct belief that you are physically and mentally able to perform the task or *self-efficacy*).

4. Ask anyone else present if they would also like a drink (language production, social awareness, compassion, recognising, strengthening and conforming to social roles).

5. Get up from the chair and walk (ability to transfer from a sitting position to a standing position, postural control, range of motion in joints, gross coordination, and bilateral integration).

6. Know where the kitchen is and how to get there (memory, topographic orientation, recognition and spatial awareness).

7. Know what steps you need to take to make a cup of tea (planning, sequencing, retrieval from procedural memory, reference to your culture and traditional way of making tea).

8. Recognise the kettle, its type and how to operate it (visual processing, figure ground discrimination, retrieval from procedural memory).

9. Fill the kettle with enough water to make the right amount of tea (stereognosis or ability to recognise an item from touch, kinaesthesia or recognition of movement, depth perception, hand eye coordination, fine coordination dexterity, grip strength, appropriate use of force, using judgement, flexibility in adapting the task for the amount of water required on this particular occasion).

10. Switch on the kettle and wait for it to boil, or light the gas on the hob and place the kettle in situ (fire safety awareness, risk awareness, sequencing, and patience).

11. Gather the cup, spoon, teabag, sugar and milk (multi-tasking, categorisation, memory of how the environment is organised, attention and divided attention).

12. When the kettle has boiled, put the teabag in the cup and pour the hot water in (hearing, interpretation of sound as a cue, safety awareness, muscle strength, exercise tolerance, timing).

13. When the tea has brewed to your particular taste, remove the teabag, add sugar and milk (decision making, self-expression, fine motor movement, hand eye coordination, memory, concentration, appropriate termination of activity).

14. Return to your chair with the cup of tea and enjoy it (lifting, carrying, judgement on pace of movement, stability when mobile, ability to perform stand to sit transfers and align self with chair).

When viewed by an occupational therapist, making a hot drink can tell us what difficulties a person is having in performing their occupations and this will begin to develop our theory or *formulation* about what is happening for that person from an occupational perspective. The assessment can also help with a possible diagnosis or what problems might be causing the difficulties. Different types of conditions might cause difficulty in different occupational performance components , so for example, someone with anatomical changes to their hands due to arthritis may have difficulty with fine motor movement and grip, someone with depression may have difficulty with initiation, motivation, concentration and dividing attention, whereas someone with memory problems may have difficulty with topographic orientation, memory of how the environment is organised, sequencing, risk awareness, initiation, divided attention and problem solving. The type of condition might make us as therapists focus on specific performance components more than others, but each person with a condition is different and the holistic assessments in occupational therapy puts the person at the centre of our formulation.

We can also extrapolate to other areas of function or other areas of life that might also be affected by that particular problem, so if someone has difficulty making a cup of tea due to arthritic changes in their hands they might also have difficulty with meal preparation, getting washed and dressed, writing, cleaning their home, and gardening etc. As a profession we also focus on what someone is able to do already, their strengths, skills, values, interests, self-beliefs, knowledge experience and realistic evaluation of their own ability, and use these as a starting point to treat the person rather than the issue in isolation.

Another key skill in occupational therapy is adapting or *grading* an occupation so that it helps someone to be independent doing it. This involves using the occupation in a therapeutic way, so we might grade the activity to address problems, or assess for what equipment would help someone to perform the occupation independently. For example if someone previously enjoyed gardening but is now unable to use tools due to anatomical changes in their hands, we might adapt the occupation to use tools that are easier to grip, or we might adapt the environment to grow more in pots where there is less digging, raking and weeding needed so that they can continue to do what they enjoy doing.

If a person is unable to perform the occupation independently, we might facilitate access to some help that would allow them to successfully complete the occupation, and here we would be assessing their potential to learn and adapt, their ability to collaborate with others and communication needs. In the above example, we might help the person to find a gardener they can work with who can complete the parts of the task they can no longer manage.

2. The importance of meaning in occupational therapy

Another key concept in occupational therapy is *meaning*. By this I mean that we are all different and have different skills; experience, values, beliefs, environments, roles and relationships, routines, aspirations, cultures, spiritual beliefs etc. What is meaningful to one person will not be to another person in the same way, and this forms the basis of our distinction between an occupation and an *activity*. Activities are the things we might do that have little personal meaning to us and therefore have little therapeutic value. We also recognise that the *purpose* of doing something is important and can add to the meaning that someone ascribes to an occupation. For example, I once worked with a client who had fallen and now had a fear of falling that was stopping her from doing her everyday occupations. She had become reluctant to walk or even stand from her chair and through this inactivity, her muscles had become weak and her legs were shaky and this coupled with increased anxiety added to her belief that she was going to fall again. She had undertaken exercise sessions in physiotherapy in the parallel bars but was not progressing well. By forming a therapeutic relationship with her, I started to ask about her *occupational history*, routines, values, beliefs, roles, home environment, and goals in the context of her culture, and to develop a

formulation about what was happening for her and how I could help.

The formulation included some of the following information:

- The clients' fear of falling was being triggered when she stood up from her chair. Her spouse was helping her up and was putting both of them at risk of injury when doing this however, as they were not using appropriate manual handling techniques.

- She was married and she and her spouse had historically had their own roles which made for a successful relationship.

- Her inability to perform her roles was making her increasingly worried about the stability and future of her relationship with her spouse.

- As she had learnt from her mother, she was the cook in the home and this formed part of her care giving role and gave her a sense of achievement and pride.

Based on this, her goal became to make lunch for her spouse. We used the therapy kitchen where I could grade the activity, manage risk of falls, coach and provide feedback in a controlled but familiar environment. Engaging in an occupation rather than the activity of exercising in the parallel bars meant that she was able to focus on the purpose of what she was doing to overcome her fear of falling. She successfully made a hot drink and sandwich during the session and she then shared the first lunch she had made for several months with her spouse. An important element of this treatment was reintroducing routine and re-establishing roles as, when life events set us adrift, these are what anchor us and remind us of who we are.

3. Occupational therapy and health promotion

The above is an example of how occupational therapy can work for people who are recovering from illness, accident or injury, however in the last 60 years of practice occupational therapy has started to move away from just a treatment of illness and towards a focus on preventing ill health, or *health promotion*. This involves the prevention of ill health (primary health promotion or *upstream* interventions), the idea of full recovery from illness (secondary health promotion) and the idea of recovering a quality of life despite living with symptoms of chronic ill health (tertiary or *downstream* interventions) and occupational therapy with its focus on holistic health and well-being, skills and strengths, and adaptation is central to all approaches at all levels of health promotion.

To most people the word recovery will relate to getting better or healing from an illness, however, in the field of chronic illness, the term is now starting to mean something different. When I refer to recovery in this resource, what I mean is the idea that someone can live well with their illness. For many people with a chronic illness they may not be free of their symptoms for any significant amount of time. This idea, at least initially, can be very difficult for some people to accept, as to give up hope of being symptom free can mean giving up hope of a cure. However, recovery is not about giving up hope, but redefining what we are hoping for. Learning about an illness, what triggers it, what changes we can make to keep ourselves as well as possible, how we can plan for the worst days, how we want to be treated when we are acutely unwell and how people will know when we are ready to take back any relinquished responsibility can gives us renewed hope for an illness which is managed better and not as catastrophic for our life journey. This concept of recovery has been widely taken up by health professionals working in the area of mental health and fits extremely well with occupational therapy. The World Health Organisation (2012) write: "*From the perspective of the person with mental illness, recovery means gaining and maintaining hope, understanding of one's abilities and disabilities, engagement in an active life, personal autonomy, social identity, meaning and purpose in life and positive sense of self*" and occupational therapy can provide all these benefits and more.

The Royal College of Psychiatrists describe recovery themes; "*Common themes in recovery include the pursuit of health and wellness; a shift of emphasis from pathology and morbidity to health and strengths; hope and belief in positive change; meaning and spiritual purpose of distress; service support reconceived as mentoring not supervisory; identity explored as a cultural issue; social inclusion (housing, work, education and leisure); empowerment through information; role change; self-care; awareness of positive language use in framing the experience of illness; personal wisdom encouraged in professional practice; and creative risk taking replacing overcautious risk assessment*" (Care Services Improvement Partnership, Royal College of Psychiatrists and the Social Care Institute for Excellence 2007) and again occupational therapy covers many of these areas in everyday practice.

However, I do not feel that the concept of recovery is understood solely in terms of acute psychiatric issues. Most of us will have experienced a life changing event that we have had to recover from, such as a bereavement, divorce or severe illness. The way we respond to this is a process of recovery, or adapting to something that will not get better, and meaningful activity, roles and routines play a key role in how we adapt to life after significant change.

The World Health Organisation (2018) writes that mental health promotion involves actions that improve psychological well-being. Godfrey (2000) writes about the role of occupational therapy in health promotion *"Because occupational therapists are concerned with occupation, they are in the unique position to observe and to influence the interplay between the individual and his or her social/physical environment and the impact of these interactions on individual and community health"*. Scriven and Atwal (2004) also point out that health promotion has been a familiar concept in occupational therapy since the 1960's and that in the 1980's the American Occupational Therapy Association advocated for the expansion of occupational therapy in health promotion. I have written this resource to be used at any of these areas of health promotion but if you are using it to recover from a significant illness or to improve quality of life with a chronic illness, please seek advice from you GP, or other health professional and get support if you require it.

4. Therapeutic occupations for mental health and well-being

Finlay (2004) writes that occupation has intrinsic value;

- As a learning tool

- By providing us with an awareness of our capacity for competence, control and mastery

- By stimulating our senses

- By structuring our time

- By meeting our needs of being purposeful and creative

- By allowing us to express and explore our feelings

- By providing pleasure through play, social interaction and connection

From my clinical practice in mental health, I have found that some types of occupations are more effective in mental health and well-being and these are based on key ideas from both the literature on occupational therapy and the wider evidence base. Below I present the key ideas and touch on the evidence base for each of them. I then describe how we can use these key ideas in a model by choosing occupations that incorporate them into a theory of health and well-being promotion to achieve a better balance of occupations that includes those that will help us to remain well, recover from illness, and achieve a better quality of life.

A. Occupations that help us connect with others

Having meaningful social connections and roles with others can promote our health and well-being. Occupational therapists believe in the concept of *social* well-being which means that the person has the opportunities, skills and knowledge to connect with others in the right amount of quality relationships that they require to maintain their well-being. In mental health and well-being, one issue that can accompany a mental health problem is social isolation, which can occur due many factors including the stigma that surrounds mental ill health, problems with confidence and self esteem, and problems with motivation and planning. In mental health therefore, occupations that promote positive social connections will generally improve mental health and well-being. However, this is not an issue just for people with a mental health diagnosis but for everyone. Increasingly in society we are moving away from opportunities to form meaningful social contacts. We can withdraw money without going to a bank teller, shop in a supermarket without going to a person on the checkout, shop online without going into a shop, spend time on social media without

seeing people face to face, text or send an instant message rather than chat in person or on the phone, and are more likely to work out of area, move away from the area that we grew up in to follow employment, use a supermarket rather than shop locally, have our own car rather than use public transport, holiday abroad, and not know our neighbours. Social isolation is also a major issue for people in later life who have further barriers to social contact with mobility issues, loss of roles, bereavement and many other factors, and this has recently been recognised in national initiatives to tackle loneliness in the UK.

Two models that conceptualise the relationship between occupation and health and well-being, identify a person's social environment as important. The Model of Human Occupation (Keilhofner et al 1980) describes the environment as the physical space, physical resources, social groups and occupational demands, including cultural conventions that the person performs their occupations in. The Canadian Model of Occupational Performance (Fearing 1997) sets the person and the occupation within the physical, institutional, social and cultural environment.

A new key idea that is gathering momentum in the occupational therapy forums is the idea that the profession is well placed to lead in the area of social prescribing. The Ways to Well-being service in York is a social prescribing service led by occupational therapist Jasmine Howard, and has demonstrated a 30% decrease in GP appointments by people accessing the service. Social prescribing recognises that a person's health is determined by social, economic and environmental factors as well as medical issues, and is aimed at addressing people's need for social contact to improve their health and well-being. Social prescribing involves medical professionals referring patients to non-medical community based support and services and examples can include, sports, volunteering, befriending, gardening, arts, and healthy eating initiatives. Paul Cooper (RCOT professional advisor) highlights the importance that any prescribed activities are genuinely meaningful to the person, in line with the key ideas in occupational therapy of occupation as central to health and well-being.

Looking outside the occupational therapy literature, The 5 Ways to Well-being initiative developed by the Department of Health in England and endorsed by the National Health Service (NHS) identifies that connecting with family, friends, neighbours and your community is beneficial for health and well-being as these can form the basic stable structure to our lives. The mental health charity Mind also attributes increased psychological resilience to performing activities that promote well-being and build social connections.

If we apply this to a model, then we can look for opportunities to connect with others when thinking about what we do in our everyday life. However, it's important for you to consider what the right amount of social contact is for you and if you are currently achieving it to your satisfaction. If you are feeling socially isolated, then this can be detrimental to mental health and well-being, but also consider the quality of the relationship as difficult relationships can also be stressful and negatively impact on health and well-being. Everyone is different and the journey through this resource is about finding out for yourself what you need to improve your health and well-being. The 5 Ways to Well-being initiative also encourages us to give to others to improve our health and well-being, volunteer our time, thank people, join community groups and contribute to our community, and ideas around taking our projects further to increase social contact are incorporated into the projects in this resource.

B. Occupations that help us to connect with nature

Another key concept in the models of occupational therapy is the *environment*. Models in occupational therapy describe the dynamic relationship between the person, the occupation and the environment, so a change in the environment can affect the person's health and well-being. By environment we mean all aspects of where we are placed, such as: the physical, social, political, institutional, organisational, and cultural environment. In mental health I have found that the natural environment can be therapeutic and there is some evidence from the literature to suggest why this might be the case. Unruh, Smith and Scammell (2000), performed a small qualitative study where three women with breast cancer who garden were interviewed, and the interviews analysed for themes. Emerging themes on the value of gardening included:

- Promotion of interactions with living things, both other people and nature.

- Meeting personal needs (creativity and challenge, preserving memories, and feeling satisfied with achievements).

- Reflections about life (rhythm to life, death and regeneration, control.

- Coping (release, escape, control and relaxation).

They conclude that *"Embedded in these garden interviews were also reflections about meaning that had a spiritual dimension. Some of these reflections concerned the life process, especially issues about controllability, one's place in life, and confrontation with mortality...The present study suggests that leisure occupations which are highly meaningful and* *may have a spiritual dimensions for the individual, enable experiences of control and stress reduction"*. Although this is a small scale study, many people who like to garden will relate to the themes that emerged.

In a systematic review of the literature carried out in 2015, ten papers over a seventeen year period were analysed to explore the contribution of allotment gardening to health and well-being (Genter et al 2015). The papers covered people with mental health issues, people in later life, allotment gardeners, parents and refugees. The main themes that emerged were;

- Allotments can encourage social connections through sharing skills, thoughts, produce and time (although the majority of the studies were carried out on organised allotment groups and this may not be the case in other settings).

- An allotment is a stress relieving environment as it is relaxing.

- Active gardening facilitated a healthier lifestyle by providing opportunities to get fresh air, access to fresh produce, and engaging with meaningful work that improved health and a sense of well-being.

- Creating an opportunity to connect with nature that could provoke an emotional response.

- Allotment gardening encourages a sense of self development and enhanced skills e.g. concentration and self confidence.

The authors concluded that allotment gardening had a positive impact on health and well-being both for therapeutic groups and for everyday allotment gardening.

Looking outside of the occupational therapy literature, The 5 Ways to Well-being also encourages us to notice the environment around us to make changes to our health and well-being. A Nature and Well-being Act. A Green paper from The Wildlife Trusts and the Royal Society for the Protection of Birds (RSPB) is a proposed piece of legislation to rescue the natural environment and its biodiversity for the benefit of people and wildlife. Nature based therapy or *ecotherapy*, has at its core the belief that we are connected to and affected by our natural environment. The mental health charity Mind are strongly advocating for the use of nature in promoting mental health and well-being and in their report Feel Better Outside, Feel Better Inside, and the authors write:

"Ecotherapy is more than going for a walk in the park or mowing the lawn in the garden. It is a regular activity that is: facilitated and structured, focused on doing an activity rather than 'health', takes place in a green environment, is related to exploring and appreciating the natural world, happens over time and involves contact with other people. Ecotherapy can improve everyone's health and well-being. Its flexibility means that services can meet a variety of needs: as a well-being service that can help everyone look after their mental health; as an early intervention service targeting people at higher risk of mental health problems, and also as services to support recovery for people with existing mental health problems."

However, I would also argue that the ideas from ecotherapy can be usefully applied to health promotion for people to maintain their mental health and well-being to prevent them from becoming unwell. Mental ill health can be related to high levels of stress and lifestyle factors, and if we perform meaningful activities in the natural environment that relax us, support healthy eating, help us to connect with others and provide some exercise, this will act as a protective factor in illness prevention. If we add this idea into our model then we can look for occupations in our everyday life that give us opportunities to connect to the natural environment to benefit our health and well-being.

C. Occupations that help us to be creative

This is based on the idea that creativity is good for our health and well-being. Cassou and Cubley (1995), write: *"The creative process is enough. It is not only enough, it is a doorway into a direct experience of the essential life force which is at the root of the urge to create art. It is the process itself-in the creative energy it releases, in the new perceptions it brings, in the deepened connection with oneself it fosters-that is at the heart of the desire to paint. To make this the whole point of painting is a simple yet radical act."*

Creativity and mental health and well-being are linked in the occupational therapy literature. An analysis of 23 peer reviewed articles published between 2000 and 2008 provide us with good evidence to suggest that creativity in occupations is beneficial to our health and well-being when the authors conclude *"Results suggest that the use of creative arts occupations in therapeutic practice may have important qualitative value related to health and well-being. Six predominant outcomes were most frequently identified across the studies; enhanced perceived control, building a sense of self, expression, transforming the illness experience, gaining a sense of purpose, and building social support"* Perruzza and Kinsella (2010).

Dynes (1989) used creative writing exercises in a rehabilitation setting for clients in a psychiatric day hospital. The rolling group programme was found to help clients talk about their emotions, feelings and ideas which helped form the therapeutic relationship. Many clients carried on creative writing after discharge from hospital. Reynolds (1997) conducted a study on the therapeutic value of needlecraft. The sample was of 35 women who described themselves as having a disability or chronic illness since their teenage years. The sample was self selecting as the researcher wanted to interview people who already did needlecraft. Themes on how this occupation was therapeutic that emerged from the interviews included; preserving or regaining a satisfactory self-image and sense of achievement and competence, coping with anxiety and depression, maintaining/enhancing positive social relationships, coping with an uncertain future, coping with pain and restricted mobility and structuring time.

Again, adding creativity into our model should help us to get the benefits to our health and well-being through our choice of occupations.

D. Occupations that help us to be mindful

This is based on the idea that mindfulness is good for our health and well-being. Mindfulness has recently become a key part of treatment for mental health and well-being, as well as being practiced by people to reduce stress and give a better quality of life. Jon Kabat-Zinn developed the Mindfulness Based Stress Reduction Program which is a psychological intervention based on meditation practices linked to our knowledge of neurological responses. *"In 1979, Jon Kabat-Zinn recruited chronically ill patients not responding well to traditional treatments to participate in his newly formed eight-week stress-reduction program, which we now call MBSR. Since then, substantial research has mounted demonstrating how mindfulness-based interventions improve mental and physical health—comparably so to other psychological interventions"*. Put simply, and in terms of how we relate the therapeutic value of mindfulness to the projects in this resource, mindfulness is about noticing what's going on around us and the sensations in our bodies rather than paying attention to the thoughts in our mind. Mindfulness has been endorsed by the NHS and mindfulness courses are now available in primary care, aimed at reducing symptoms of stress, anxiety and depression.

The 5 Ways to Well-being also advocates for mindful practice in everyday life to enhance health and well-being and encourages us to be curious, notice the beautiful, savour the moment and reflect on experiences to help you to appreciate what matters to you. (The last way to well-being, learn is also incorporated into this resource, both in trying new occupations and taking them forward by finding opportunities to learn more in the future, whether this is talking to others, reading around a subject, researching on the internet, or taking a course).

In occupational therapy, I feel that there is a good comparison to be made between the concept of mindfulness and the idea of *flow*. Flow is a phenomenon that occurs when the demands of an activity precisely match the abilities and interests of the person, enabling a person to get fully engaged and absorbed in an occupation. When in a state of flow, the person is not being distracted by thoughts and there is a relief from symptoms of stress, anxiety and depression.

To demonstrate the therapeutic use of occupations that are mindful, creative and that help us to connect with others and with nature to promote health, I'd like to give an example of how I use baking to help myself recover during an episode of depression. For me, baking is about creativity as I like to experiment with recipes and when I am well I find I can lose myself in the process of baking or achieve flow and often look around in surprise when I'm finished to find a very messy kitchen! Creativity when I'm unwell can help my thoughts become a bit freer. Baking is also a way in which I care for and nourish myself and other people in my life. When I'd started to feel a little better after being unwell recently, I decided to bake. Making decisions can be really difficult when someone is depressed so this was definitely a step in the right direction and I noted that. I then decided on a basic scone recipe, another good start and set goals around making some scones to share with my friend when she visited the next day to say thank you for her support during my illness.

Planning skills can be affected by low mood, so writing out the ingredients that I needed and where I could get them was a good opportunity for me to start doing this again, it also ensured that I didn't forget anything because low mood makes me forgetful. Going outside can feel overwhelming when I am unwell so I will tend to avoid it, but I needed to go out to buy the ingredients so that gave me the motivation to do it. I usually have to bargain with myself that I'll just make one trip then stay in for the rest of the day. To go out I had to shower and put on clean clothing, style my hair and put a little makeup on, something I hadn't done for a while and it felt good to do that, I felt more like "me" because I looked more like my usual self. I went out and intentionally went to the smaller shops in my town, which meant I had to speak to shop assistants a little. The exercise was also nice as I'd not been very active for a while. Being out helped me to notice the weather and that it was sunny on that day.

Having bought the ingredients I found all the equipment I would need and organised it on the worktop. I started to make the scones, measuring out the ingredients and using my judgement from knowledge and experience. I also started to decide on the flavours and went outside to my blueberry bushes to pick some fresh fruit. It was warm in the garden and I searched for the best fruit, feeling the sun on my face. I had to concentrate whilst I made the scones, something else that can be difficult when I have low mood.

I rubbed the butter into the flour, feeling the texture with my hands. I smelt the vanilla essence as I added it. I kneaded the dough, cut out the scones and put them in the oven to bake, setting the timer in case I forgot what time I had put them in. I could smell them baking and started to get a little hungry which was something I hadn't felt for a while. I also started to feel like "a baker" again. The scones turned out really well and I felt a sense of pride when I tasted one still warm from the oven. I realised that the morning had past and I was now tired but more relaxed and could rest for the afternoon. In this one occupation I had been creative, social, mindful and had connected with nature, I had exercised, practiced cognitive skills, regained some sense of self, structured my time and made a caring gesture in the role of friend.

5. The therapeutic use of self compassion

One of the key themes to emerge from my work with people with mental health difficulties and in my own recovery journey is the idea of the therapeutic benefits of having compassion for others and for one's self and this is another idea I would like to draw into our model. The concept of giving to others in the 5 Ways to Well-being can also be helpfully included here, as the concept of giving to others is linked to health and well-being, but it does not consider self-compassion as important. Drawing from ideas from Eastern philosophy, Buddhism, evolution and neurology, Paul Gilbert writes: *"We can stimulate patterns in our brains that are self-nourishing, supportive, encouraging and soothing, so that in whatever we do to help ourselves (say, change the way we think about ourselves or face up to and cope with things we struggle with), we practise creating in our heads an experience (brain pattern) of warmth, kindness and support as our primary starting position. If we do this, we may find that things will be slightly better for us".*

This just means for our model of practice we start this journey by being gentle and encouraging with ourselves. We develop curiosity to try new things and a belief that what we produce is good enough and not to be compared unfavourably with others. We can treat ourselves and our creations as we would treat others and try and leave behind self-criticism of the steps we take. Mistakes are part of learning something new so if something doesn't turn out how we would have liked, we have learned what not to do.

6. Health and well-being through therapeutic activity: An Occupational Therapy Informed Model of Health Promotion

Bringing together all the key points and ideas from occupational therapy, health promotion, and self-compassion, below I have illustrated what the ideas above look like in terms of understanding how everything fits together and is understood in this resource.

We start with the person and everything the person is as an occupational being, with their occupational history, values, beliefs, skills, knowledge, relationships, roles, aspirations, and spirituality that make up their personal meaning or what is important to them. By spirituality I don't mean just religious beliefs. Spirituality for me is connection with nature, and it's my feelings of being in the right place or exactly where I should be at that time, but spirituality will mean different things to different people. However, it isn't essential to have a sense of spirituality or religious beliefs to benefit from this model.

When thinking about what we can do to improve our health and well-being we start from a position of having compassion for ourselves and not judging what we do negatively. We are nurturing and giving ourselves permission to try something new in a safe environment by being encouraging with ourselves.

We then look for activities that are meaningful (occupations) and help us to be more social, more mindful, more creative and connect with nature, and build these into our routine to achieve more balance in the things we have to do and the things we want to do to improve our health and well-being. The routines can become a lifestyle aimed more at promoting our health and well-being. Our lifestyle will then support us to understand ourselves or our occupational identity, and help us develop the skills, knowledge, and self-efficacy (our belief that we can achieve what we want to). By using the natural environment, we can improve health and well-being, and by choosing occupations that help us to make more social connections, we can develop our social environment so we have the amount of meaningful social connections that is right for us.

The model is dynamic as the more we understand ourselves, develop our skills, increase our knowledge and have more belief in our abilities, the more confident we are at developing the occupations that will maintain and improve our health and well-being and try new things. However, the aim is not to have more and more occupations over time, but enough to

give balance to your daily life so you are replenishing yourself (or keeping you bucket topped up) and developing resilience towards life's challenges and the demands on your personal resources. When our demands are balanced with our resources, we might call this a state of equilibrium. We might also develop into teaching skills to others in particular areas. As we age, we change, and some occupations will change as well, so there might be occupations that you no longer engage in, or that you intend to go back to and some that replace others. We might need to adapt some occupations to our physical ability as our bodies change in later life. We might also have times when we have more freedom to do the things we want to do, upon retirement for example, and health promotion through occupational therapy will help us to adapt to changes, structure our time, be mindful for health, stay connected to the natural environment, maintain our skills, fulfil our roles and stay fit and healthy with a good social network so we do not become isolated after our worker role has ended.

Health and well-being through therapeutic activity: An Occupational therapy Informed Model of Health Promotion

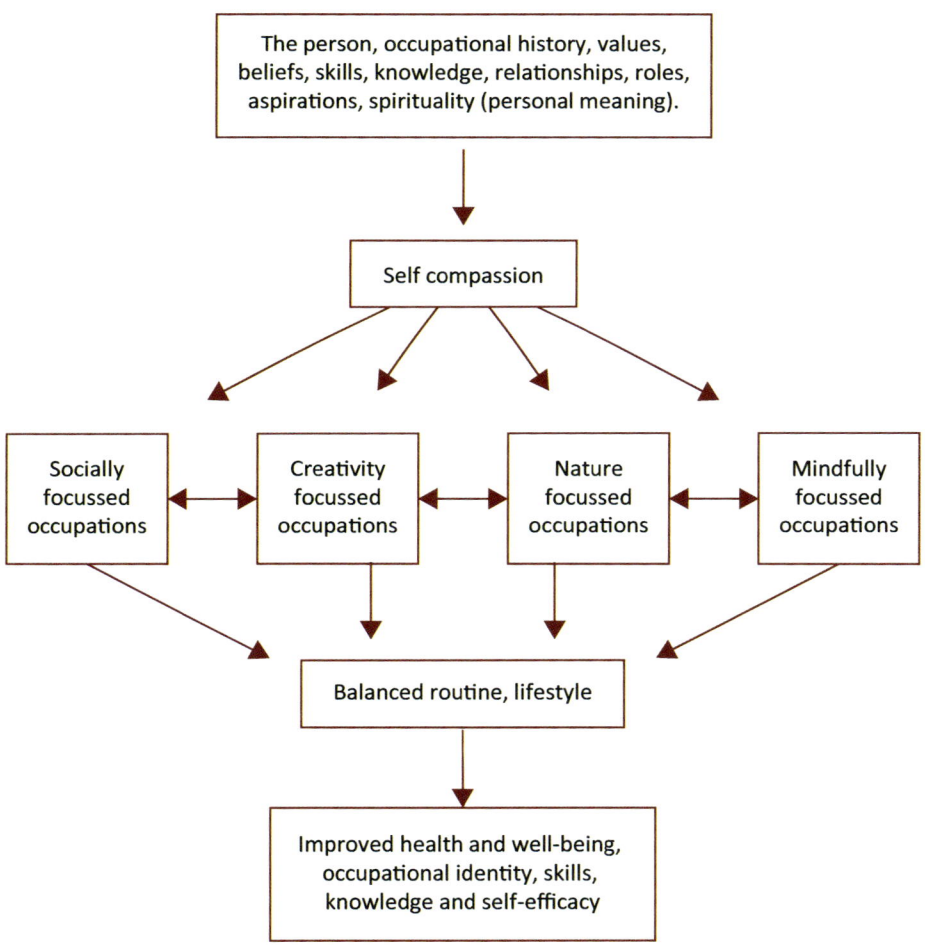

7. How to use this resource.

- Keep a journal

"Writing in a journal reminds you of your goals and of your learning in life. It offers a place where you can hold a deliberate, thoughtful conversation with yourself."

– Robin S. Sharma

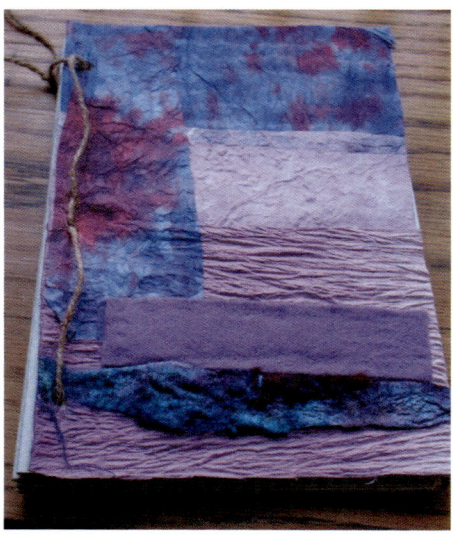

I'd like to suggest that you either make or buy yourself a notebook that is small enough to easily take out with you to record reflections, ideas, recipes, art work, stick in special objects, inspirational pictures, poems, website addresses, sketches, photographs, or anything that you might find useful that comes out of the different projects in this resource. This is your journal and there is no right or wrong way to do it. You might prefer to write notes or make it more visual, or abstract, whatever is meaningful to you. I decided to make mine by using some old watercolour paper, folding it in half, hole punching it, making a front and back cover with decoupage pattern using up some different colour papers, and threading some string through, securing with a knot.

Other ideas for your journal.

- Rate your mood

You might find it useful to measure how you are feeling at the start of your journey, at the beginning of a project and straight after finishing it, and at high or low points along the way. Use a rating scale that is quick and easy and you are more likely to do it, such as marking on a scale of 1 to 10 where you are at this moment, with 1 being very low in mood and 10 being very happy in mood. **If you feel distressed by any mental health symptoms, please see the resources section at the back of this book to find support.**

- Make a weekly schedule

	MORNING	AFTERNOON	EVENING
MONDAY		*Buy baking ingredients*	*Baking for Jane's birthday tomorrow*
TUESDAY			*Jane's for celebratory catch up and homemade cake*
WEDNESDAY			
THURSDAY			
FRIDAY			
SATURDAY		*Walk in the park to collect leaves and write in nature diary*	
SUNDAY	*Harvest veggies, find soup recipe and shop for extra ingredients, make soup*		*Craft night with the girls-soup and leaf printing Christmas cards*

Block out time to do the projects that you want to try or supporting activities. Try and prioritize some time for yourself to enhance your health and well-being as sometimes we need to give ourselves permission to do this. In occupational therapy we use the diary system for *behavioural activation,* which means that having a daily schedule can help you to see your work life balance, how you spend your time, and start to do new things, as you have specifically put aside time to do this and the labels act as a cue for action. If we want to improve our health and well-being, one of the most powerful ways we can change behaviour is to incorporate health and well-being time into our routines so that it becomes our lifestyle and we do things to support this automatically.

- Goal setting

Goal setting is used effectively in occupational therapy to allow a person to recognise how far they have come in treatment. I also use goal setting myself to motivate myself to do things. Try to set some goals for each project using the SMART method and this will help you to be successful in achieving them;

> Specific (exactly what are you going to do?).

> Measurable (how will you know when you've achieved the goal?).

> Achievable (is the goal within your capability or do you need some help?).

> Relevant (is the goal something that's meaningful to you and will it help you get to where you are aiming for?).

> Timely (what timescale are you giving yourself to complete the goal?).

Examples of smart goals:

By the end of this week I will have collected enough blackberries to make four fruit crumbles for my friends.

Take it forward

This relates to thinking about the next steps on your journey. This resource aims to provide some initial ideas that will signpost you in the directions you can take to further your engagement in the occupation after you have completed some of the projects. Decide if and how you would like to take the ideas forward and write these in your journal. This is to help you to structure your time and make the activities into occupations that you "do" rather than "have done once".

- Make it more meaningful

Make a section in your journal to explore what is personally meaningful to you. Here are some questions that might help you reflect on this that were inspired by models in occupational therapy (The Model of Human Occupation (Kielhofner et al 1980), The Canadian Model of Occupational Performance (Fearing et al 1997), and The Kawa Model (Iwama 2006).

- What was your favourite subject at school and why?

- What did you want to do when you grew up?

- If you work, or have worked, what did you like about what you did?

- If you work, do you feel you have a good work life balance, and if not, what is stopping you from achieving this?

- What are your main strengths?

- What roles do you currently have in your life and which are the most important and why?

- What's your greatest achievement so far?

- What was the best time in your life so far and why?

- What are you good at?

- What do you do already that makes you feel better?

- What do you do that makes you happy?

- What's important to you?

- What have you always wanted to try or get better at?

- Who do you most admire and why?

- What culture or cultures do you most identify with?

- What do you wish you had more time to do?

- What do you hope to get out of this journey?

- What religious or spiritual beliefs do you hold?

- Where do you most enjoy going to on days out?

- What couldn't you live without?

- If you won the lottery tomorrow, how would your life change?

- What do you value most about where you live?

- If you could live anywhere in the world, where would it be and why?

- How do you care for yourself?

- How do you care for others?

- Who are you closest to in your life and who can you go to for support?

- What groups do you belonged to?

- What issues are you passionate about?

When you have done this exercise, start at the beginning of the book and:

1) Read through the project

2) Consider what is meaningful to you and how you can tailor the project to this meaning. For example with the Bake chapter, think about the following questions:

- Do you remember cooking at school or when you were a child and did you enjoy it?

- Did you ever go fruit picking when you were younger?

- Did anyone bake for you when you were younger?

- Can you bake this for someone to show gratitude for something they have done for you, or just to be kind?

- What is culturally meaningful for you to bake or use as a specific ingredient?

- Would you like to make more home cooked food to support a healthier diet?

- Have you got friends or colleagues who bake that you can chat to about recipes?

- Have you baked before and did you enjoy it?

- Is baking something you would like to be better at or something

you are generally proud of when you have done it before?

- Is baking fun and relaxing for you?

- What kind of baker are you? One who enjoys the accuracy of measuring and timing, or one that starts with a recipe then thinks they can improve it?

3) Consider which "Make it" options you want to add in to make it more focused on creativity, nature, connecting with others or mindful.

4) Set your SMART goals.

5) Determine what resources and materials you will need and gather them.

6) Rate your mood on the scale from 1 to 10.

7) Do the project.

8) Rate your mood again and notice the difference.

9) Reflect in your journal if this type of project is something you want to do more of and if so, block some time in your weekly schedule.

10) Take one of the given examples or think of your own way of taking your interest further in the future.

CHAPTER 1

Bake

"Cooking and baking is both physical and mental therapy"
– **Mary Berry**

1. Autumn fruit crumble

This is a lovely warming crumble for those cold autumn days and one of my favourite recipes. If you haven't baked before, this is a good one to start with. I remember making apple crumble at school and proudly carrying it home.

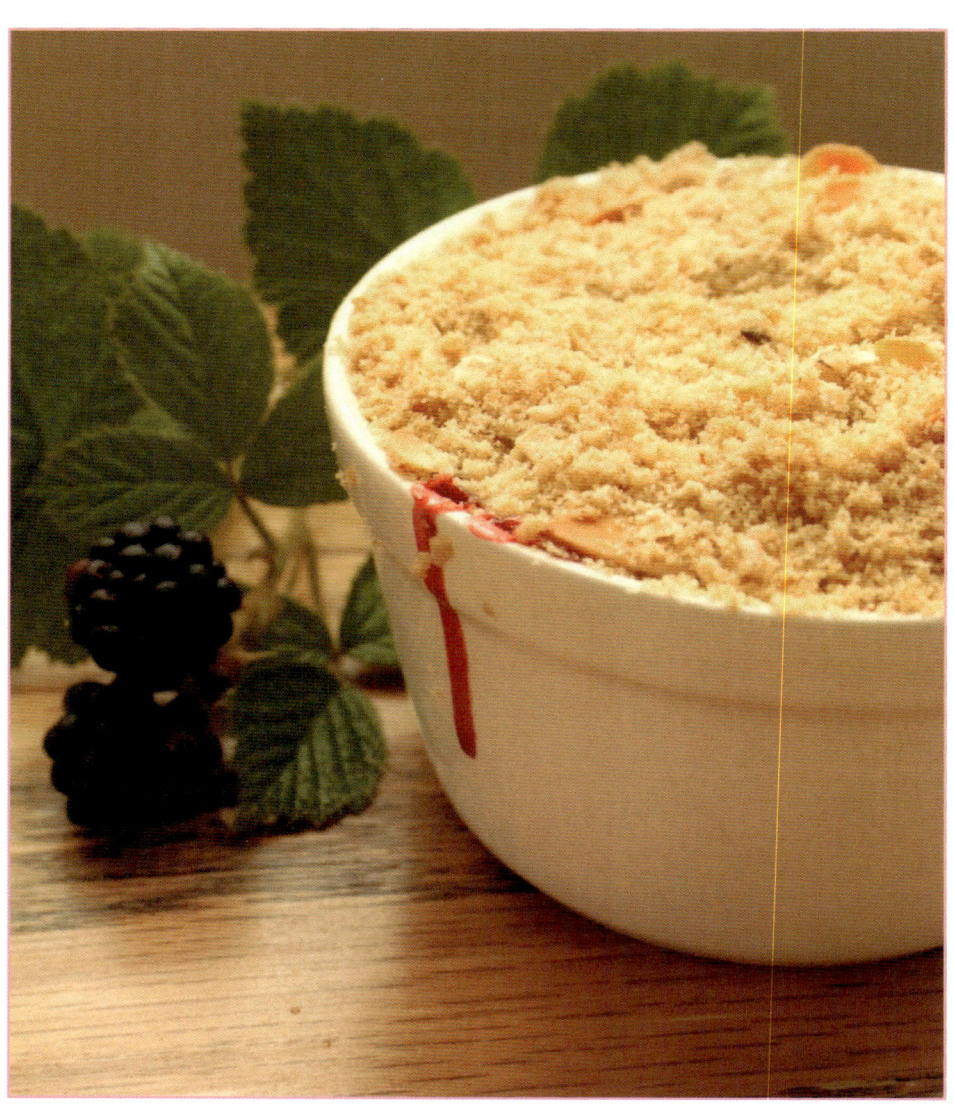

Ingredients you will need:

- 250g (grams) of blackberries
- 700g (approximately four large) ripe pears
- 200g plain flour
- 100g unsalted butter cut into cubes
- 40g flaked almonds roughly chopped
- 40g rolled oats
- 100g caster sugar
- 100g Demerara sugar

Equipment you will need:

- Kitchen weighing scales
- Four individual ovenproof ramekins 4 inches in diameter
- Large mixing bowl
- Mixing spoon
- Knife
- Chopping board
- Large saucepan
- Large spoon or ladle
- Baking tray

Method:

- Preheat the oven to 190⁰C (170⁰C fan, or gas mark 5).
- Wash the blackberries well.
- Peel the pears, cut out the cores and chop into cubes of approximately 1cm square.
- Put the pears into the saucepan over a medium heat and add the caster sugar, cook for approximately 10 minutes until the sugar is melted and the fruit begins to soften, then add the blackberries, return to the boil and cook for 1 minute then remove from the heat and spoon the mixture into the ramekins.
- Put the flour and butter into a large bowl and rub together with your finger tips to combine until it looks like breadcrumbs. Stir in the sugar, chopped almonds and rolled oats. Hold each ramekin over the bowl and sprinkle a generous amount of crumble over the top. Put the ramekins onto the baking tray and place on a shelf in the centre of the oven. Bake for 25 minutes or until golden brown on top. Enjoy.

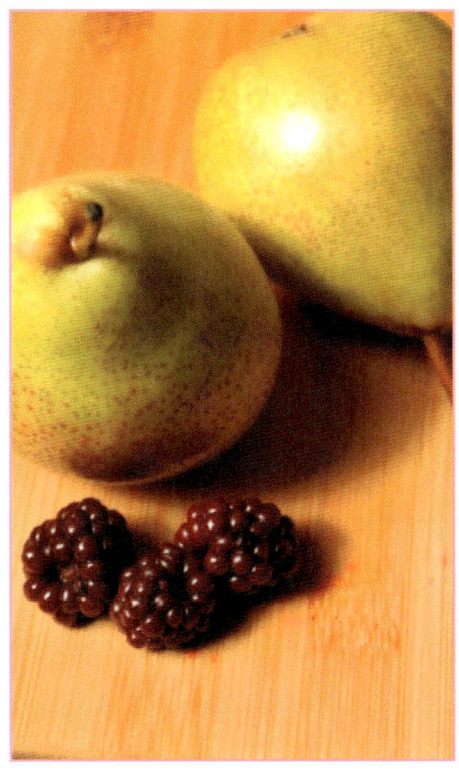

Make it more social

One of the ways we can recapture a sense of community is to get to know the people in our neighbourhood, so instead of going to a supermarket, purchase your ingredients from local shops and take the time to chat to people.

Invite some friends over to share the crumble or go for a walk together to pick berries.

Bake with a friend or family member, or teach your children as you go.

Blog your activity or just a photo of what you make and share it on social media.

Ask friends or relatives if they have any traditional recipes they can share with you.

Connect with nature

In blackberry season, take a container and head outdoors to pick fresh fruit. Take your time to notice where brambles are growing in public areas, such as your local park or area of hedgerow. You can freeze the berries in batches if you need to pick over several days by washing and drying them, laying them on a baking sheet on a tray so they don't touch each other, and when they are frozen transfer into a container or freezer bags and store in the freezer until you need them. If you have space, grow your own fruit.

Make it more creative

Be curious about how you can adapt this recipe to your own taste.

Use apples instead of pears, follow the recipe as above.

Use 500g of frozen mixed berries instead of pears (blueberries, raspberries , strawberries) cook on the hob with the blackberries and sugar for 3 to 4 minutes (reduce this time to 1 to 2 minutes if using fresh berries) or until the sugar has melted and the fruit starts to release its juice. Continue as basic recipe above.

Add the recipe to your journal and take photographs or make illustrations of your crumble, add tips and ideas for the next recipe.

Serve with cream, ice cream, custard or vanilla yoghurt

Make it more mindful

Slow down and notice the smell of the ingredients as you chop them, the fruit as its cooking, and of the baking crumble. Notice the feel of the butter and flour as you work it into a breadcrumb texture. Notice the taste of the finished crumble. Can you identify the different textures as you eat or any of the individual flavours?

If you are picking fresh berries, notice the different colours of the ripe, ripening and unripe fruit. Find the ripe fruit and pick, taking care to avoid thorns. Taste some of the fruit. What can you hear whilst you are picking the fruit and can you identify each different sound? What can you smell? How do the berries feel between your fingers?

Take it forward

You could find and enrol on baking course. Use this link to find further education courses in your area https:// nationalcareersservice.direct.gov.uk/ course-directory/home (there may be a cost for courses).

Find a local foraging course to keep the cost of baking down and get more exercise and time in nature. For your local foraging workshop or course, type "find a foraging course near me" into your search engine, alternatively, the Woodland Trust has lots of information so follow this link https://www. woodlandtrust.org.uk/visiting-woods/ things-to-do/foraging/. Always make sure you know what you are picking as some berries are poisonous.

Buy a baking book or borrow one from your local library and find another recipe you want to try. Schedule this in your diary. Charity shops can be a good source of cheap recipe books and is a way of helping others. You could also look online for free recipes.

11. Botanical biscuits

These pretty little biscuits are easy to make and taste great. The lemon flavour works well with the sweetness of the icing. They are crumbly like short-bread and go well with a cup of tea.

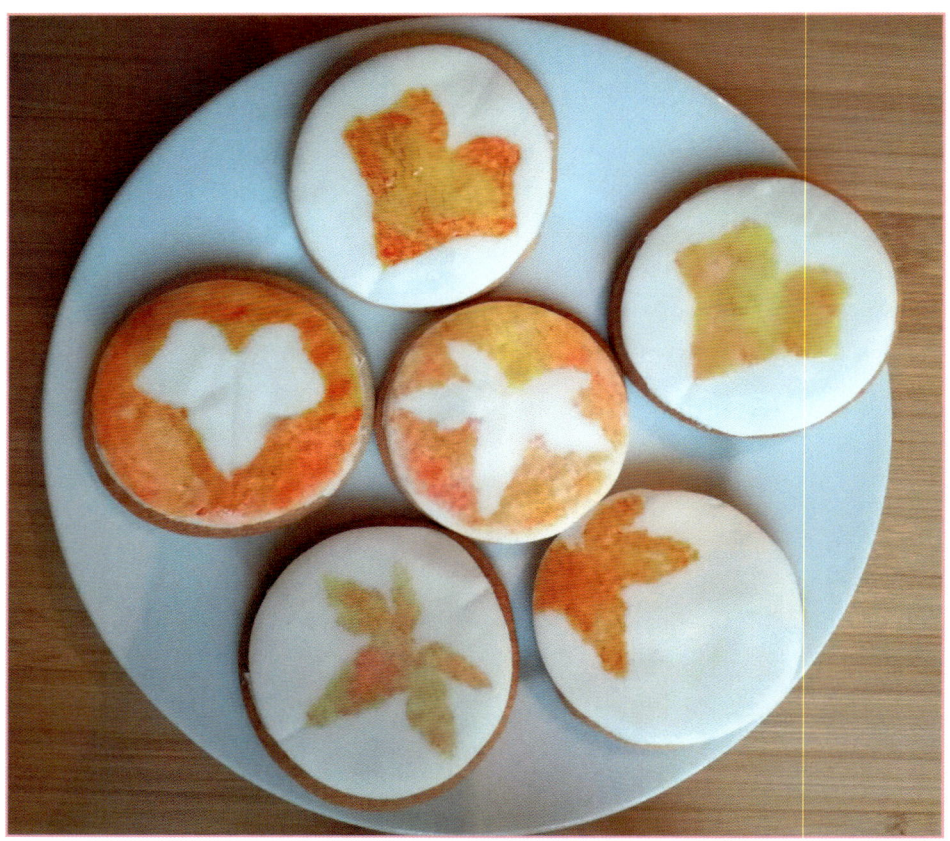

Ingredients you will need (makes around 24 biscuits):

- 200g caster sugar
- 180g unsalted butter at room temperature and cut into small cubes
- Zest of 1 lemon (this means using a grater to remove the yellow skin (zest) of the lemon)
- 1 egg
- 1egg yoke
- 320g plain flour
- 1tbs (tablespoonful) plain four to roll
- 1kg (kilogram) ready to roll fondant icing
- 1 tbs icing sugar to roll
- Yellow, red, green and blue liquid food colouring

Equipment you will need:

- Kitchen weighing scales
- Round 6 ½ cm diameter biscuit (or "cookie" cutter)
- Greaseproof paper
- New clean paint brush
- Baking tray
- Large mixing bowl
- Rolling pin
- A pair of scissors

Method

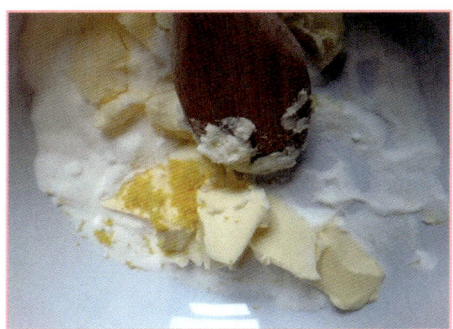

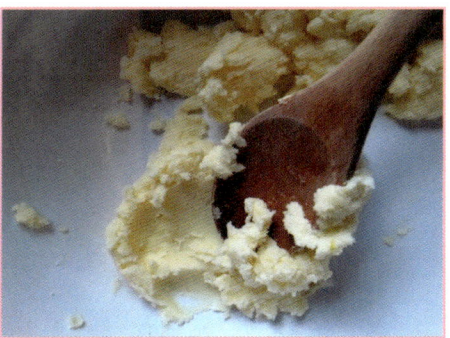

- In a large dish, cream the caster sugar, butter and lemon zest together.
- Add the egg, egg yolk and plain flour and mix until it comes together, then knead with your hands until fully combined.
- Put the dough in a covered dish and refrigerate for one hour.
- Preheat oven to 200°C (180°C fan, or gas mark 4).
- Sprinkle flour on your work surface and roll the dough, turning as you go, until it is approximately the thickness of a one pound coin.
- Cover the baking tray with the greaseproof paper and

this will stop the biscuits from sticking to the tray.

- Cut out 24 biscuits and gently transfer them onto the baking tray. They shouldn't spread out very much, but leave a gap in between each one just in case. If you don't have a large oven, you could bake them in batches.
- Bake for 10 to 12 minutes or until golden brown. Slide the paper and biscuits off the baking tray and onto your work surface and allow them to cool down.
- Whilst the biscuits cool, cut out leaf templates from the greaseproof paper.

- Sprinkle 1tbs of icing sugar onto a clean work surface and roll out the fondant icing to half the thickness of a pound coin.

- Cut out rounds with the same biscuit cutter and wet them with a little water with your finger before placing one on top of each biscuit, press down gently and smooth the edges with your finger.
- Put one or two drops of each food colouring on a saucer with space to mix colours as you go.
- Choose a template and position it over the top of the iced biscuit, patting down gently.
- With your paintbrush, dip into the colour and tap on the saucer until the brush is almost dry.
- Stipple (dab) around the edges and fill in the middle of the template

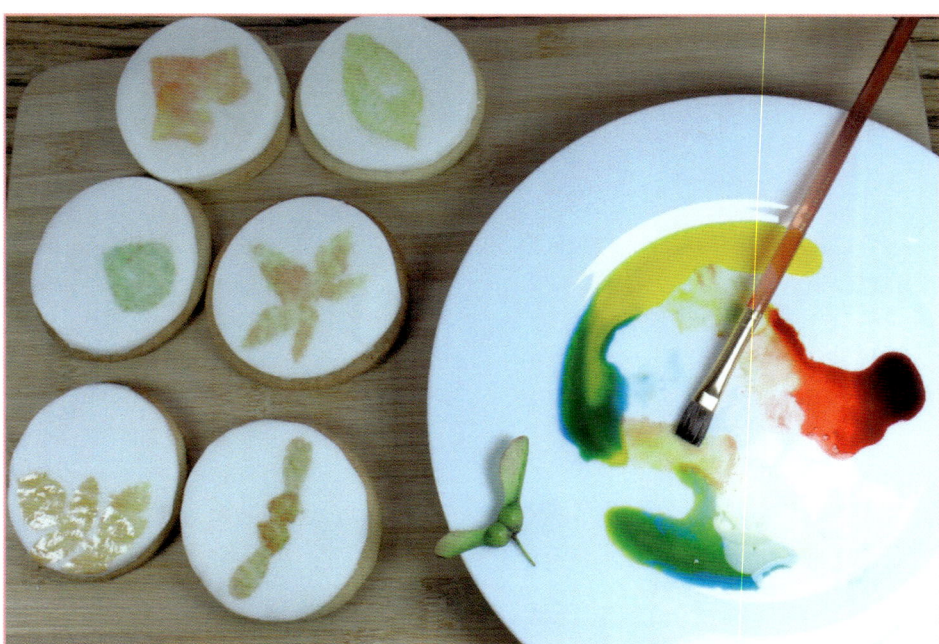

with colour. You could use just one colour or a mix of colours.

- Remove the template gently, lifting straight up so the colour doesn't smudge.
- Allow to dry over night then enjoy your botanical biscuits.

Make it more social

If you are going to walk to find inspiration for your cookies, walk with a friend or tie in the session with a walk with a walking group.

Make the biscuits to sell for a charity at work.

Make the biscuits as gifts at Christmas or for a birthday, or just to say thank you to someone. Pre purchase some patterned cellophane bags, bag ties and ribbon to add that special touch.

Take the biscuits on a group walk to share with others.

Connect with nature

Find inspiration for your templates by taking a walk outdoors. Look for as many different shapes of leaves as you can and collect one of each. Look for simple but bold shapes. Look for seeds, shells, anything with an interesting shape. Use these to inspire your templates by looking closely at the shape,

folding over the greaseproof paper and cutting out a profile of it.

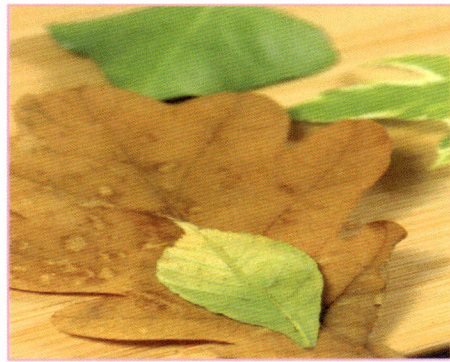

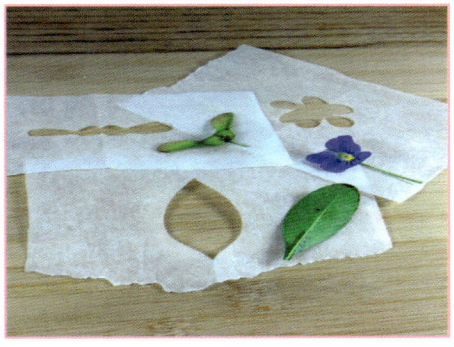

Make it more creative

Experiment with different flavours for your biscuits, instead of the lemon zest, try a teaspoonful of chopped lavender leaves, or half a teaspoonful of almond essence, or a teaspoonful of desiccated coconut. Find a recipe and make your own fondant icing, which again can be flavoured and coloured to your taste. Try different shapes of cookie cutters, place the templates in the centre of the icing, or off to one side to give a profile. Paint directly onto the biscuits instead of using templates. Use edible glitter, or edible gold leaf to accent the leaves.

Write on the biscuits with edible ink, find inspiration from images, designers, styles or photographs.

Add your favourite recipe combination to your journal and take photographs of your biscuits and add tips and ideas for the next recipe.

Make it more mindful

Slow down as you bake. Notice the smell of the lemon zest as you cream it with the butter and sugar. Does the lemon smell intensify as you work? Notice the feel of the dough as you knead it. Look in detail at the leaves you have collected if you are using them for inspiration, notice the shape and try and trace it as you cut the paper. Experiment with the colours when painting, mix them and try to match them to the colours of the actual leaves. Notice the taste of the biscuits, can you taste the lemon and does the biscuit crumble in your mouth?

Take it forward

You could find and enrol on baking course. Use this link to find further education courses in your area https://nationalcareersservice.direct.gov.uk/course-directory/home (there may be a cost for courses).

If you can make some space in a kitchen cupboard for baking supplies and look out for flavourings and decorations when you shop so you have a store of ingredients.

Visit some patisseries for inspiration.

Find some other biscuit designs you want to try such as iced Christmas biscuits to give as gifts.

Schedule in your next baking day.

III. Cheese and herb scones

This is an easy savoury scone recipe. It was the first savoury scone recipe I tried and smells amazing whilst it's cooking. This recipe makes one round that can be cut into approximately 8 individual scones.

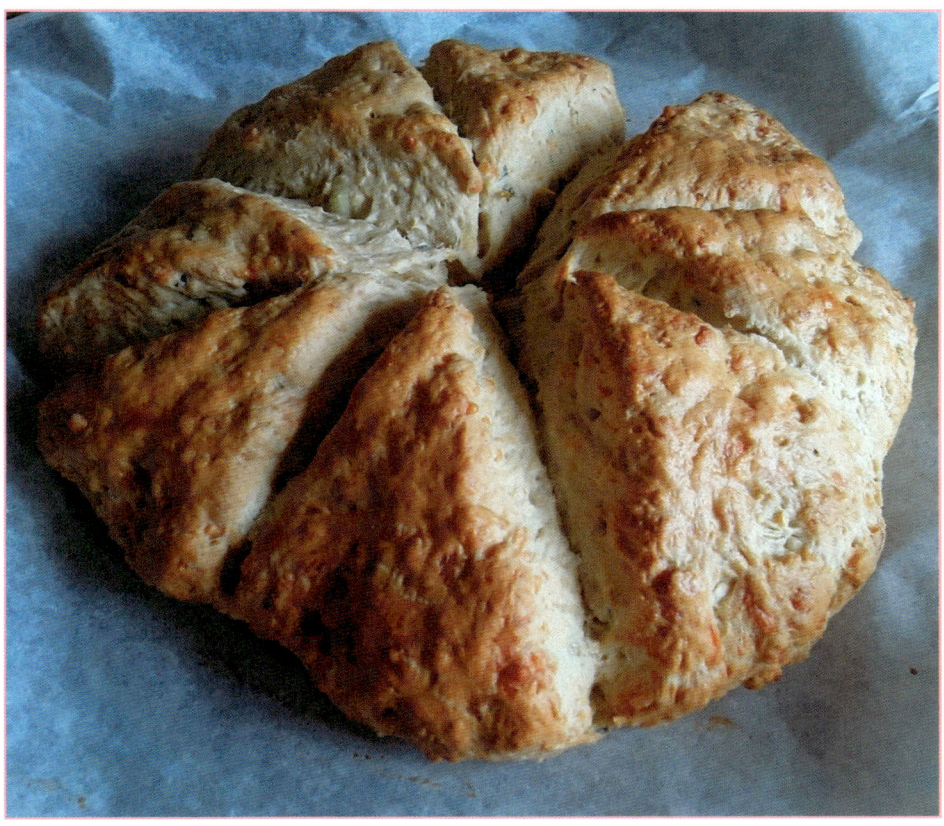

Ingredients you will need:

- 150g mature cheddar cheese grated
- 350g self-raising flour
- 4 medium spring onions trimmed with the outer skin removed and finely chopped
- 1tsp (teaspoonful) baking powder
- 1tsp light brown sugar
- 85g salted butter chilled and cut into cubes
- 1 large egg
- 150ml semi skimmed milk
- 1 tbs chopped fresh thyme and marjoram combined

Equipment you will need:

- Kitchen weighing scales
- A large mixing bowl
- Wooden spoon
- Pastry brush
- Greaseproof paper
- Baking tray
- Knife
- Jug

Method

- Preheat the oven to 180°C (160°C fan or gas mark 4).
- Line a baking tray with some greaseproof paper.
- Put the flour, sugar and baking powder in the bowl and mix it together.
- Add the butter and rub between your fingers to combine into a rough breadcrumb mixture.

- Stir in the cheese, spring onion and herbs.
- In a jug, mix the egg and milk together, beating the egg to break the yolk.
- Pour most of the egg and milk into the flour mix, but leave a tablespoonful for glazing.

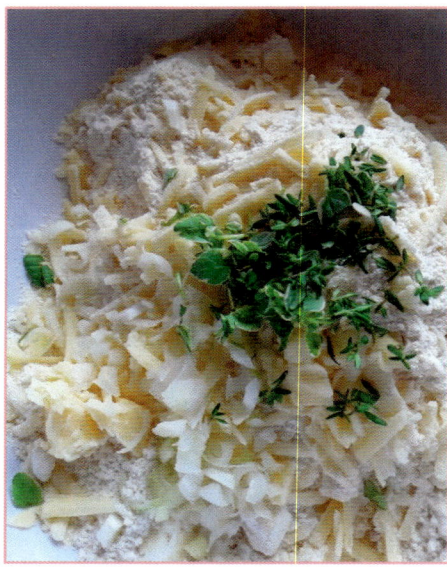

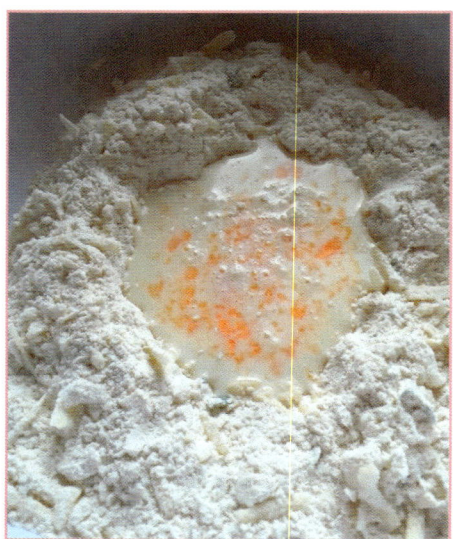

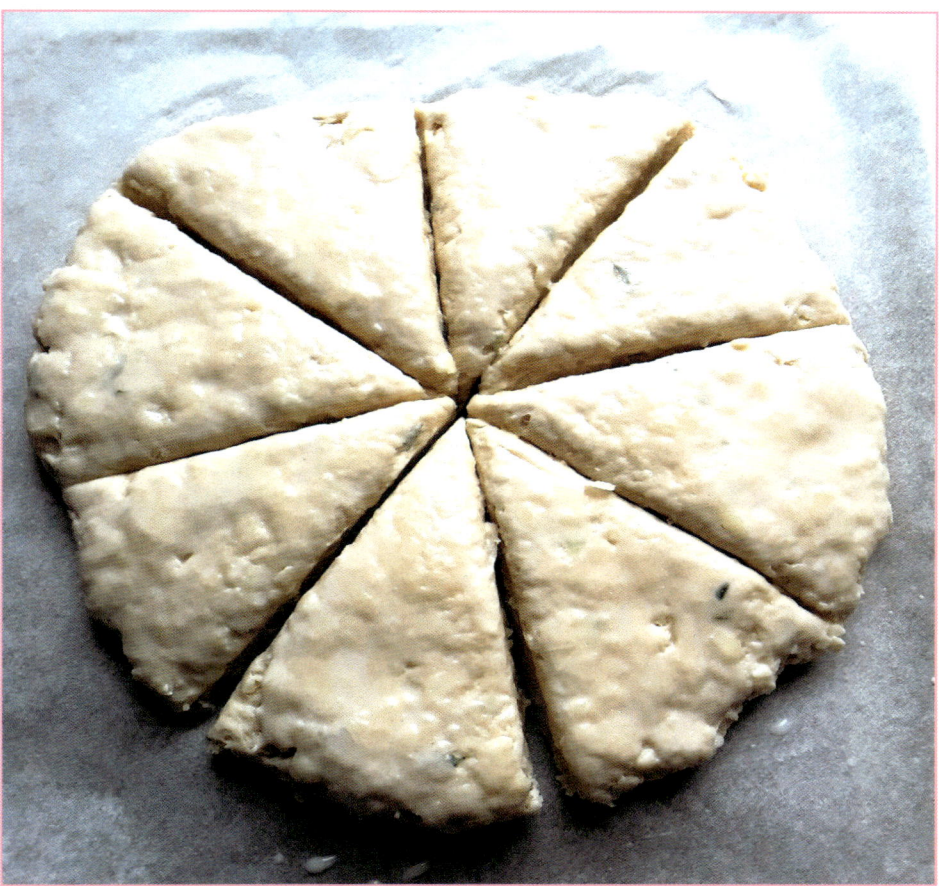

- Mix together with a spoon until a rough dough forms.
- Flour your work surface and tip out the mixture, working it until it just forms a uniform dough (don't over work it).
- Roll the dough into a ball then pat and turn it until it forms a round approximately 2 cms thick.
- Score into 8 equal sized pieces but leave the pieces in the round, this will make it easier to cut when it's baked.
- Glaze the top by brushing with the remaining egg and milk mixture.
- Bake in the centre of the oven for 25-30 minutes until the scones are golden brown. Enjoy.

Make it more social

Arrange a craft night with your friends and serve warm as a dumpling with a thick vegetable soup (see autumn roasted vegetable soup recipe in chapter 4, Cook).

Make a homemade scone and jar of chutney mini hamper as a Christmas gift or to take along to have after a meal cooked by a friend or family member (see Christmas chutney recipe in chapter 4, Cook).

Connect with nature

Grow your own herbs in teacups (see chapter 2 Grow).

Grow your own spring onions in a vegetable plot in a pot (see chapter 2, Grow).

Pick wild garlic on a walk, wash well, pat dry and use one finely chopped tablespoon in your recipe .

Take the scones on a picnic when you go for a walk.

Make it more creative

Experiment with other home grown vegetables e.g. one medium potato coarsely grated, two cloves of garlic thinly chopped, or 2 small red chillies thinly chopped (see chapter 2 Grow).

Use other home grown herbs such as marjoram, chives, basil, try mixing them all together or just add one or two.

Add a teaspoon full of cumin, ground coriander or turmeric, or half a teaspoon full of cayenne pepper.

Add your favourite combination to your journal and take photographs of your scones and add tips and ideas for the next recipe.

Find a good chutney recipe and adapt it to your taste and make to go with the scones

Make it more mindful

Slow down.

Notice the feel of the mixture between your fingers as it forms into rough breadcrumbs.

Notice the smell of the spring onions as you chop them, the smell of the herbs as you pick and chop them, and the smell of the scones as they bake.

Close your eyes and taste the fresh herbs, cheese and spring onion.

Notice the colours of your ingredients, the green herbs against the yellow cheese and white flour, the golden brown tops of the glazed baked scones.

Take it forward

You could find and enrol on baking course. Use this link to find further education courses in your area https://nationalcareersservice.direct.gov.uk/

course-directory/home (there may be a cost for courses).

Schedule in your next baking day.

Find another scone recipe to try, maybe a sweet one this time, you could try apple, raisin or cherry.

http://www.thefreshloaf.com/ has free bread baking recipes and if you can make scones, you can make bread as it's a similar process.

CHAPTER 2

Grow

"Flowers always make people better, happier, and more helpful, they are sunshine, food and medicine for the soul."
— **Luther Burbank (American Botanist)**

1. Teacup herb garden

This idea is great if you want easy access to fresh herbs to use in your kitchen. It also means that you can grow even if you have limited or no outdoor space, all you need is a windowsill.

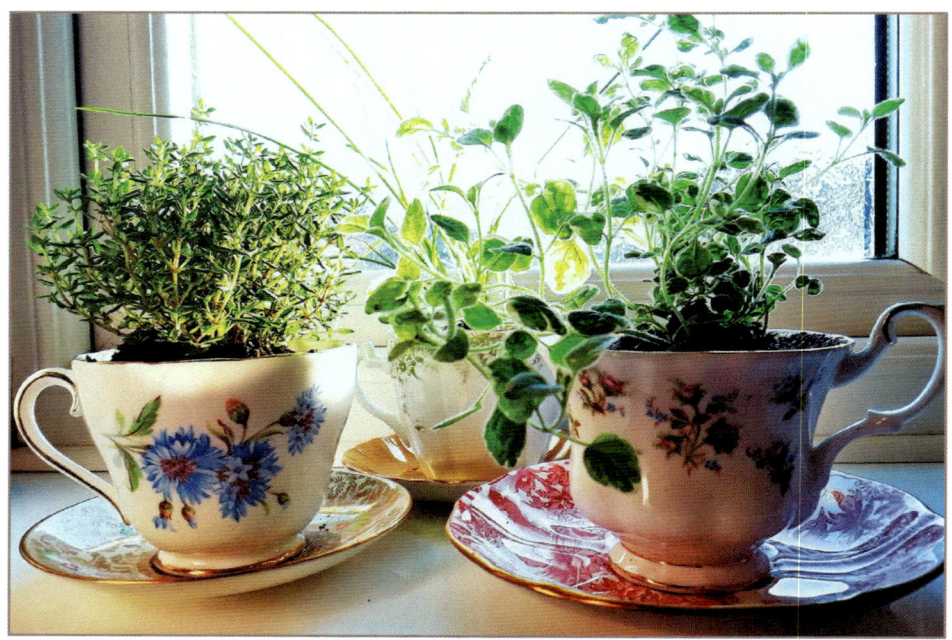

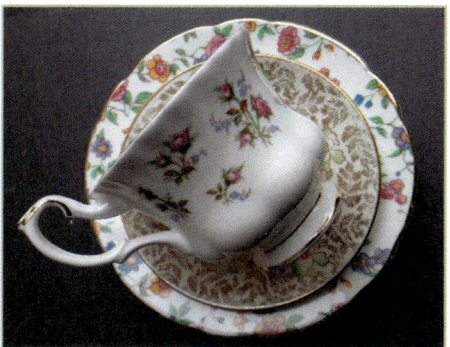

Equipment you will need:

- 3 teacups with saucers and optional side plates (mismatched is fine but avoid any with chips or cracks as they may shatter when drilling).
- Masking tape
- Electric drill with 10mm masonry bit. (If you don't have one and can't borrow one from a friend, hire shops are a good alternative and it should be relatively cheap to hire the equipment for half a day or a day. You may also need an extension lead if you are planning to work outside).
- Eye protecting goggles
- Disposable dust mask
- Some old newspaper
- Potting compost
- Thyme, marjoram and chive seeds
- Fertiliser (plant food)

Method

- Choose a dry day if you are working outdoors and find a surface to work on that is a comfortable height and stable.
- Set up your drill and choose your first cup.
- Turn the cup upside down and place a cross with the masking tape over the centre of the base of the cup, this will prevent the drill from slipping until the bit bites into the ceramic.

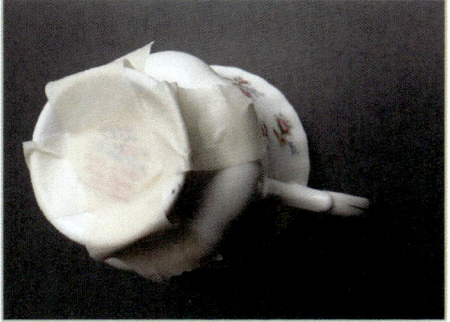

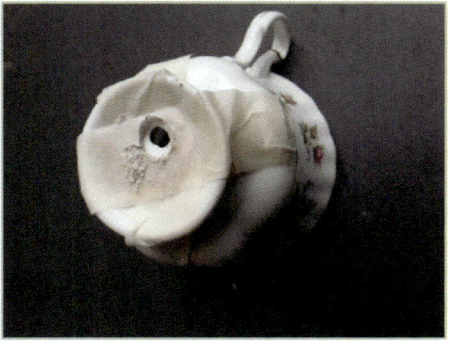

- Put on your protective equipment.
- Position your drill directly above the teacup at 180 degrees angle and starting off slowly, press down gently but firmly.

- Drilling may take a couple of minutes but keep checking and when you see the hole start to form, ease off the pressure so the drill bit doesn't go right through the hole as this can shatter the cup.
- When the hole is around 1cm wide, stop, tap the dust off the cup being careful not to touch it as it may contain sharp pieces, and tip the dust from the newspaper into a dustbin.
- Repeat for all three cups.
- Fill the cups with potting compost to approximately 1cm from the top of the rim.
- Wet the compost to remove any air until the water starts to come out of the drainage holes you have drilled.
- Sprinkle 2-3 thyme seeds onto the compost in one cup, 2-3 marjoram seeds onto the compost in the next cup, and 10-12 chive seeds onto the compost of the third cup.
- Sprinkle over a fine layer of compost to cover the seeds.
- Place on a windowsill and do not allow the compost to dry out completely.
- Feed once a week with the plant food.
- When the seedlings start to grow you may need to thin out by removing the weaker ones from the thyme and marjoram cups but leave all the seedlings in the chive cup.
- Enjoy your fresh herbs.

Make it more social

Go vintage shopping to charity shops, maybe with a friend to find your teacups or containers.

When you thin out your plants, plant up other containers for family, friends, and colleagues.

Use the herbs to make the Cheese and Herb scones in Chapter 4, Bake and the autumn roasted vegetable soup in Chapter 2, Cook and invite friends or family for lunch.

Connect with nature

Decorate some containers with pressed flowers or leaves that you have collected on a walk. Choose cups decorated with natural themes, leaves, flowers or colours that you might find in nature, greens, browns, reds, etc

Grow other herbs and vegetables in pots to cook with, see the other projects in this section.

Make it more creative

Take your time choosing your cups and saucers and mixing and matching colours until you find the ones that are just right for you.

You can use almost any container to grow in so be creative with this. A drainage hole is important so choose a container that already has one or one that is not too thick to drill or poke holes into e.g. wellies, teapots, milk jugs etc. Alternatively, make your own container from moulded concrete, polymer clay, a container that you have decorated with paint, collage, beads or yarn.

. . . .
Make it more mindful
. . . .

Connect with the nurturing side of yourself as you tend the seedlings. Can you notice when the first tips of green emerge from the dark compost? Observe how the seedlings change as they grow from the first leaves to maturity. If you crush a leaf between your fingers, can you start to smell the scent of each of the different herbs? Notice the different colours of the plants and different shapes of the leaves.

. . . .
Take it forward
. . . .

Keep picking your herbs and use in salads, infuse in oils for cooking by chopping up and adding a tablespoon full to 100mls (millilitres) of vegetable or olive oil, and chop up the herbs and put them in ice cube moulds with water to freeze in the freshness and use a frozen cube in recipes.

Herbs can be used to make Christmas wreaths and smell amazing for weeks, find instructions in a book in the library or on the internet, gather the equipment in time for Christmas and have fun.

If you have some outside space, plant some lavender seeds and use the flowers to infuse caster sugar or chop up a teaspoonful of leaves for lavender scones (see Chapter 1, Bake). Plant a mini herb garden in a pot (see below) or plant herbs in amongst your flowers or vegetables in pots (see below), or in your garden.

11. Instant spring garden in a pot

This is also a great idea for engaging with nature if you have limited outdoor space. If you have no outdoor space choose indoor plants and see the "Connect with nature" suggestion box for more ideas for indoor instant gardens. It can be planted with seeds to reduce the cost, but if you want an instant garden, use small plants.

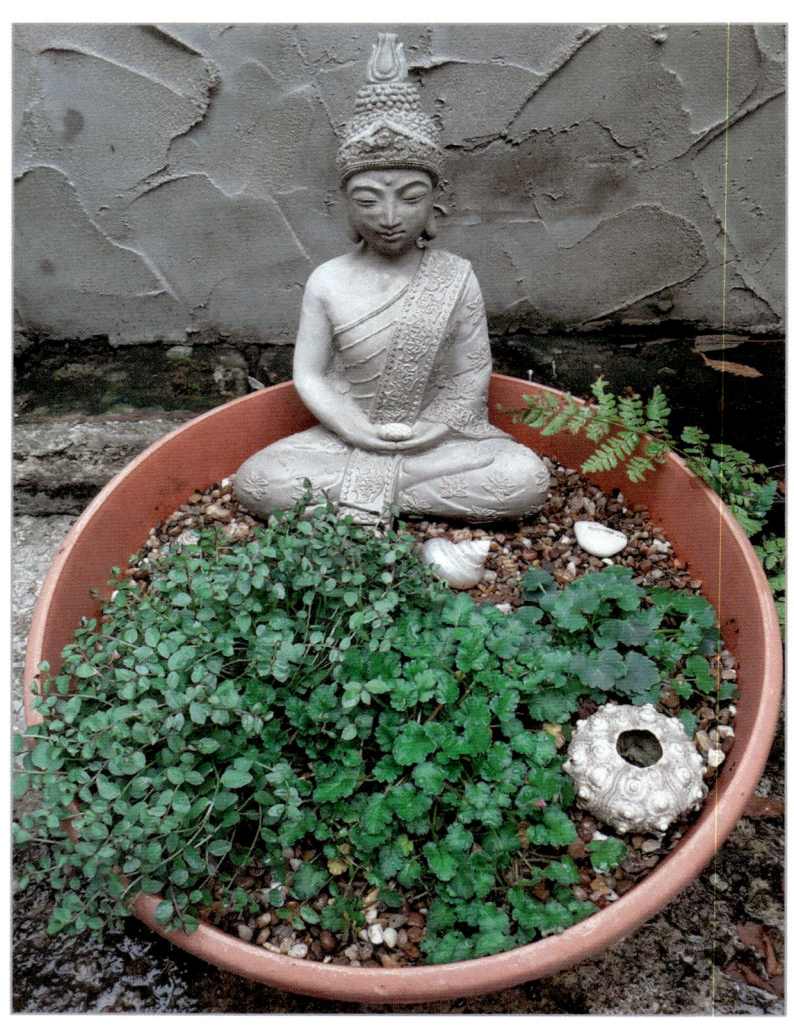

Equipment you will need:

– A container to plant in (I used a round one that already had drainage holes in)
– A dish to put under the container to catch any water if you are making your garden to grow indoors
– A selection of small plants. I used alpines for outdoors but you can use indoor plants if you don't have outdoor space. (Try and choose plants that thrive in the same type of compost and conditions as you will be planting them up together).
– Enough compost to fill up your chosen container (be guided by the advice on the plants for your choice of compost)
– A bag of small gravel.
– A handful of pebbles or broken terracotta pieces
– Decoration of your choice (I used a small Buddha inspired ornament)
– Plant food (if required in the plant care tips of the plants you buy)

Method:

▪ Put the pebbles or broken terracotta pieces into the bottom of the pot to ensure that the drainage holes aren't blocked with compost (if the plant roots sit in water, they can rot).
▪ Fill your container with the compost to about half an inch from the top.

▪ Place your plants and decoration in position on top of the compost until you have worked out your design. When you are happy with how it looks, plant the plants into the compost.
▪ Put a layer of gravel, approximately 1cm thick on top of the compost and around the base of your plants so that you can't see the compost. Place your chosen decoration on top of the gravel.
▪ Place the dish under the container if you are making an inside garden.
▪ Water in well and feed once per week or as your plant care instructions advise you.

Make it more social

Visit garden centres, plant nurseries, community allotments, community gardens and DIY stores for plants and materials for your garden. Get advice from staff on choice of plants and plant care.

Be inspired by a family member, friend or neighbour's garden and talk to them about it.

Make a mini garden as a gift for someone.

If you are new to gardening, find out if anyone you know is experienced in it and get some tips.

Connect with nature

On your walks look out for decorations for your garden, shells, pebbles, branches, anything that you like.

Choose a natural theme for your garden, for example: make a mini forest, a stream with blue coloured glass, beach with sand, hills covered with locally collected moss, Zen garden with different coloured gravel. Visit places for inspiration, take photographs or make sketches to work from in your journal.

Make a "living log" garden by finding a log with moss growing on it and hollowing out a channel to plant with succulents and locally growing fern seedlings. Decorate with pebbles, shells or anything you think compliments your planting. Notice any wildlife that your garden attracts.

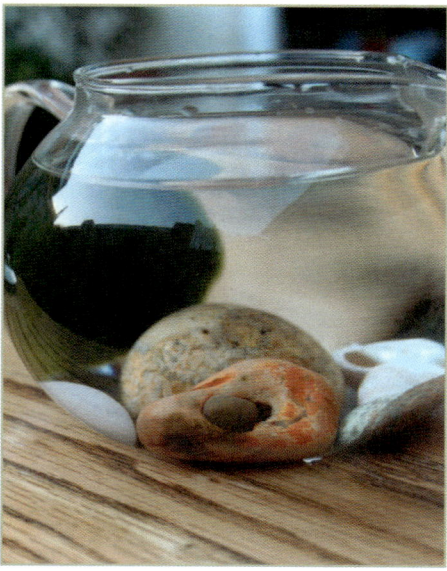

Or if you have less space, make a mini water garden in a teapot with some Marimo moss balls and your favourite pebbles and shells. Choose to use elements of a favourite place (see Chapter 3, Photograph) in your garden that bring back good memories or capture the atmosphere.

Make it more creative

Choose different colours of gravel, stone chippings, slate chippings, sand, shells or chipped bark and contrast or compliment the colours of the plants you have chosen.

Alternatively, make your own container from moulded concrete, polymer clay, or use a container that you have decorated with paint, collage, beads or yarn (remember to make it a weatherproof design if you are making it for outdoors).

Make or buy decorations for your garden, figures, houses, temples, bunting, and prayer flags whatever you like to make the garden meaningful for you and add a spiritual element if you like.

Add solar lights or candles to light your garden in the evening to give it a magical feel.

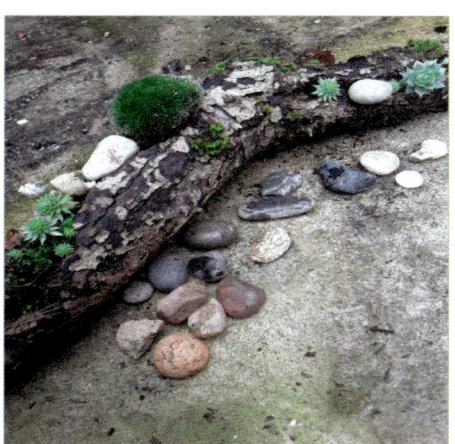

Make it more mindful

Connect with the nurturing side of yourself as you tend your garden.

Choose scented plants or herbs to use in cooking, notice the different colours of the plants or flowers, which compliment or contrast each other.

Notice the feel and the smell of the compost as you work with it.

Notice the sound of the gravel, sand, chippings or shells as you work it around your miniature garden.

Spend time noticing the changes in your garden as it grows.

Take it forward

Schedule in your next growing project.

Thrive is a charity that brings about positive changes in the lives of people with disabilities or who are vulnerable through gardening www.thrive.org.uk/. Their website www.carryongardening. org.uk/ has information on gardening for emotional well-being, gardening with a physical health issue, as well as hints and tips to remove barriers to growing.

A great way of accessing green spaces and giving to others if you haven't got a garden or allotment is to volunteer to maintain the natural areas around you. If you want to find about more about conservation volunteer opportunities information can be found at these sites:

 www.gov.uk/government/get-involved/take-part/volunteer

www.tcv.org.uk

www.wildlifetrusts.org/volunteer

www.rspb.org.uk/volunteer

III. Organic vegetable plot in pots

Growing your own vegetables can reduce the cost of grocery bills, support a healthy diet and be rewarding. Waiting times for allotments can be long and it can be hard to manage one if you have other time commitments, so why not start your own in pots. It can be taken with you if you move too.

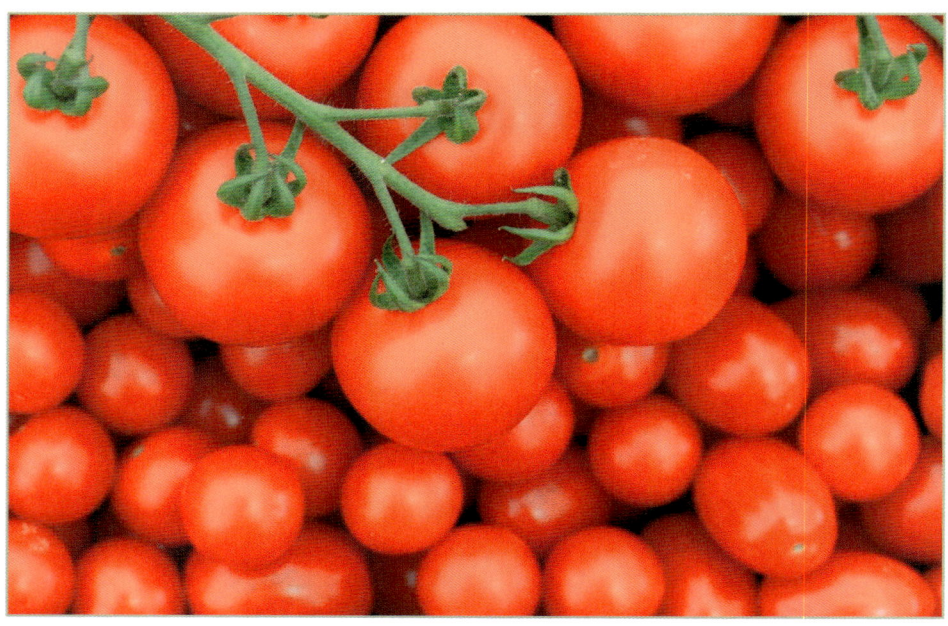

If I'm growing food to eat, I always grow organically and this just means not using chemicals or pesticides on the plants. There are lots of natural ways of managing pests and diseases but expect some damage and loss. By growing your own food you will also be getting the most vitamins and minerals from what you eat as there is less time between harvesting and eating. You can also reduce food waste by picking only what you need and care for the environment by reducing packaging.

For this project the starting point is for you to decide what you like to eat. There's a variety of vegetables, herbs and fruit that can be successfully grown in pots so start by making a list in your journal and doing some planning. Some vegetables can be grown indoors but if you have outdoor space you can grow a huge variety of produce. Next, research the varieties that are best suited to container gardening, the growing conditions you have access to, planting and harvesting information. You need to consider the space you have to grow in and it's position (shady, part shady, full sun) as plants that are positioned correctly will grow better. Do you have a yard, balcony or decking to put pots on or are you going to be using window boxes or hanging baskets? You can then gather appropriate containers and compost, pebbles or terracotta pieces for drainage, together with seeds or seedlings and fertilisers. Remember that the first cost will be the highest, but you can

be creative in what containers you grow in and reduce future cost by keeping the seeds from your plants to use the next year and starting a small compost heap in a container to turn your food waste into compost. Plastic containers are usually cheaper and lighter than terracotta or ceramic and are less likely to crack in the winter. Check websites like Freecycle and eBay for cheap job lots of containers and wash them well with hot soapy water if they have been previously used.

Below is an example of the list I made when planning my vegetable plot in pots. I wanted beetroot to make chutney with and blueberries to add to scones. I bought a blueberry plant from the garden centre and potted on into a larger pot with ericaceous compost as they can take some time to grow to the size needed for a good crop. For the other crops, as the compost needed to be well drained, I added horticultural grit to a good quality potting compost. I also needed some sturdy canes for the beans and to prop up netting to deter birds and cats.

	Variety	Position	Soil	Plant	Harvest	Fertiliser
Tomatoes	Gardeners delight	Full sun	Well drained	Mar-April	When ripe	High potash
Beans	Dwarf French	Partial shade	Well drained	May	Jul-Sept	Well rotted manure
Beetroot	Mini beet	Full sun	Well drained	Mar	Jun-Oct	General purpose
Squash	Courgette	Full sun	Well drained	May-Jun	Aug-Sept	General purpose and high potash when fruit
Onion	Garlic	Full sun	Well drained	Oct-Nov	May-Jun	General purpose
Spinach	Nagano	Shade	Well drained (grow under bean plants)	Apr-Sept	Perpetual cut and come again	General purpose
Brassica	Kale	Partial shade	Well drained	Apr-May	Oct onwards cut leaves as needed	Nitrogen rich
Blueberry	Sunshine blue	Full sun sheltered from wind	Ericaceous Water with rain water	Nov-Mar	Jul-Sept	Nitrogen rich

The Royal Horticultural Society website has lots of information on gardening, choosing plants, pests and diseases etc that you don't need to be a member to access. Follow this link to find out about growing your own vegetables.

www.rhs.org.uk/advice/
grow-your-own/vegetables

Make it more social

My neighbour and I share some communal space at the back of our homes and when I asked if she would mind if I put some pots there to grow vegetables, she was really interested and we decided to make it a joint venture.

My local allotment society holds open days where they sell produce, seeds and bulbs and I go along to increase my stock and get tips or advice. Check if your local allotment society or community garden does something similar.

Connect with nature

By tending your pots you will spend more time outdoors. Try and set aside ten minutes a day to water and weed and put this on your schedule. Notice any changes in weather to decide what to pick before the first frosts of the year. Notice any insects and wildlife attracted by the crops and look up any you don't know the names of.

Visit kitchen gardens open to the public for inspiration.

Make it more creative

Try unusual varieties and different crops, be curious about what you can grow and don't worry if it isn't successful, it's a learning process about the conditions you have.

Plant edible flowers in amongst your crops to support your cooking.

Experiment with all the space you can find to grow and improvise containers.

Make it more mindful

I tend to work the compost with my hands and notice the feel and earthy smell of it.

Look for signs of seedlings starting to grow and change, look carefully for signs of pests or disease, notice the produce ripening, smell and taste it.

Take your time deciding what to gather and cook, then cook mindfully (see Chapter 4 Cook).

Take it forward

If you decide to get an allotment, The National Allotment society provides lots of information related to allotments and finding one near you, as well as growing advice, advice on planning an allotment, monthly jobs in the gardening year, composting, organic growing, and pests and diseases

https://www.nsalg.org.uk/.

Apply for an allotment via this link https://www.gov.uk/apply-allotment just put in your postcode and you will be directed to you local council website.

A community allotment can be a good way to grow produce and meet people as well. It is managed by a group of people, so takes less time and commitment than having your own allotment. Type "community allotment near me"

into your search engine to find your nearest projects.

Why not think about starting your own community allotment. Follow this link for funding sources

https://assets.publishing.service.gov.uk/government/uploads/system/uploads/attachment_data/file/7594/2203634.pdf.

The RHS also put on annual flower shows around the UK that can be great for inspiring you to grow. Take a camera and snap ideas for later, you can also buy seeds and plants and chat to other gardeners. The RHS also have information on courses and workshops that you can get involved in for a cost https://www.rhs.org.uk/.

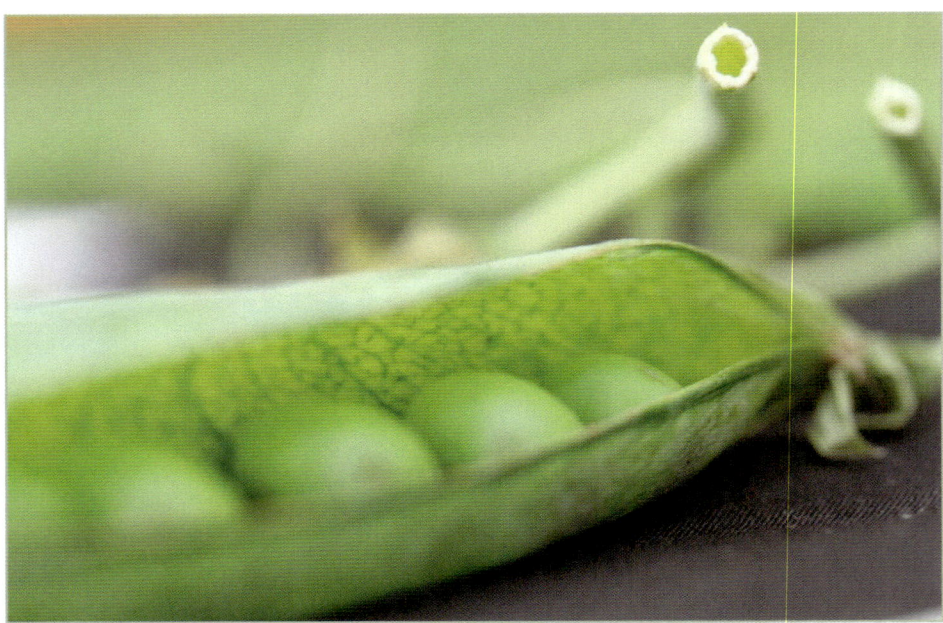

CHAPTER 3

Photograph

"*I love this life. I feel like I am always catching my breath and saying, 'Oh! Will you look at that?' Photography has been my way of bearing witness to the joy I find in seeing the extraordinary in ordinary life. You don't look for pictures. Your pictures are looking for you*".

– Harold Feinstein

1. Mindful photography walk

By noticing what is around us, we become mindful of our surroundings. Mindful photography can help us to focus, concentrate, express ourselves creatively and be curious. I have used mindful photography as a therapeutic tool when working with people with depression and anxiety as it helps to focus the mind on the environment rather than on anxious or negative thoughts.

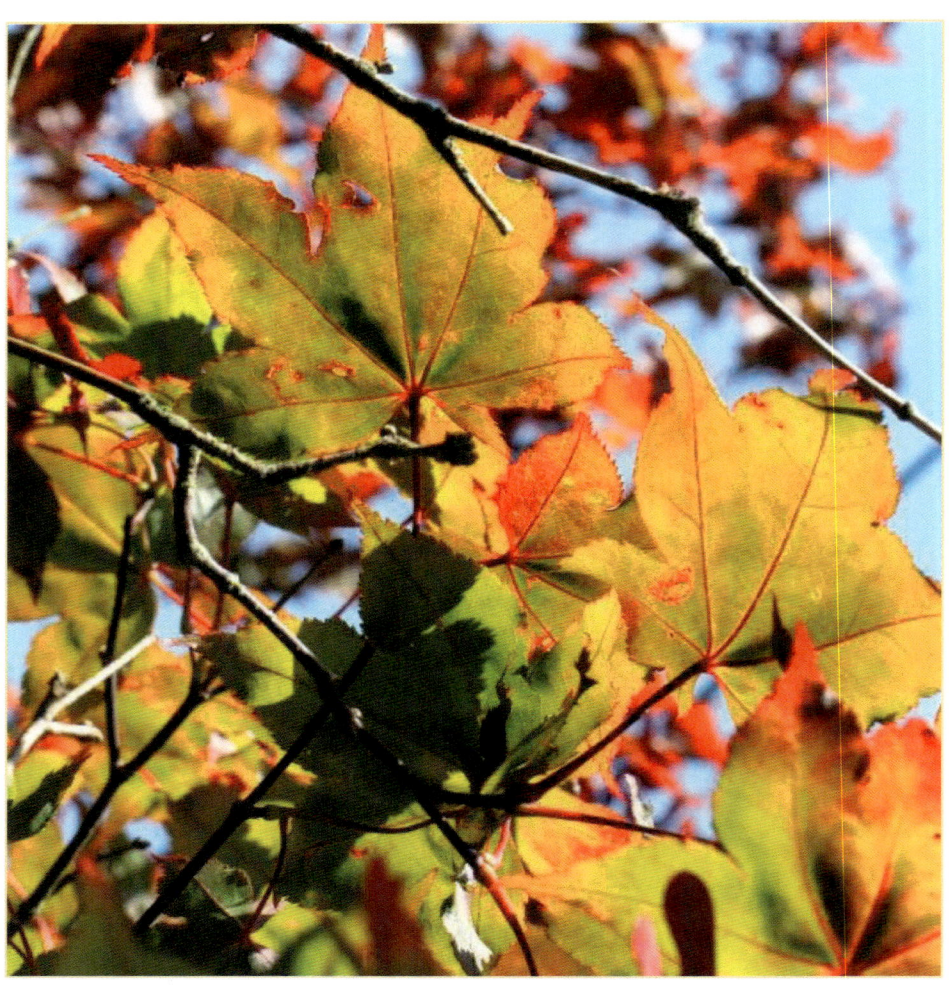

Mindful photography is a great way to slow down and really notice the world around us and can add therapeutic value to a walk. This project is based around mindfulness and nature, but there are still ideas on how to make it more social and creative below.

Method

- You do not need an expensive camera for this exercise as most mobile telephones now have a camera. If you do not have access to a camera, simply use the prompts below as a nature scavenger hunt and notice the objects, ticking them off your list.

- Plan a walk in a park or in the countryside and follow the prompts below. Don't worry if you can't find everything, it's more important to take notice, so we are concentrating on the process and not the outcome. If you are using a camera, try and take a nice photograph of what you find to use in projects later.

- Find something that is unique.
- Find something that smells amazing.
- Find something that feels smooth.
- Find something that feels cold.
- Find three different types of leaf.
- Find two different types of seeds.
- Find three different coloured flowers.

- Find a bird by following its song.
- Find something that reminds you of another place.
- Find something you think is beautiful.
- Find a rock that looks like something else.
- Find something that makes you smile.
- Find something that is heart shaped.
- Find something that is a home for something else.
- Find a natural mandala (a center with a pattern radiating out).

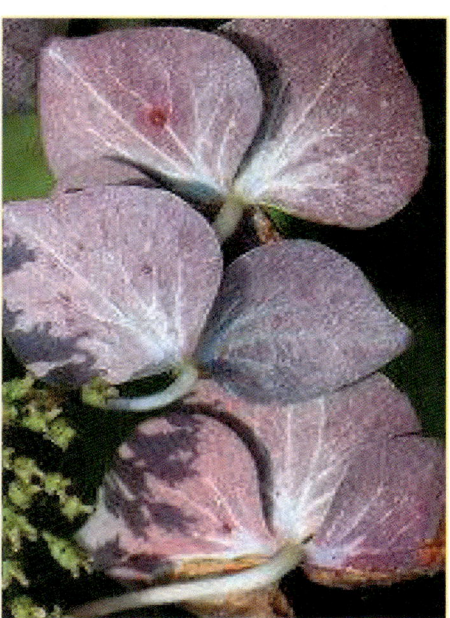

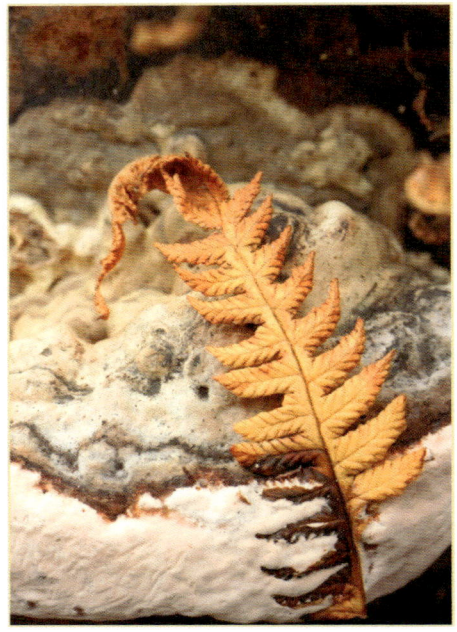

Turn your photographs into greetings cards.

Make it more creative

Find something you can use to make a gift for someone.

Use your photographs for inspiration for cutting out stencils for your Summer Botanical biscuits in Chapter 1, Bake.

Use your photographs for inspiration for nature inspired textile pieces, perhaps one for each season (see Chapter 5, Craft)

Make it more social

Invite someone along on your walk and lead your own mindful walk.

"Meetup" is an international organisation that was set up to help people to connect after the 9/11 terrorist attack in America. The website allows people to set up interest groups and find other people with similar interests. Groups are usually free or at a nominal cost to cover administration charges. See if there is a Meetup photography club in your area, register and sign up for it.

On your walk find something to give to someone else that will make them smile.

Take it forward

Schedule in your next mindful walk.

The National Trust is a charity for places of historic interest and natural beauty in the UK, follow this link to find out more

https://www.nationaltrust.org.uk/ and it is free to search for places to go on days out but there may be an entry cost. The National Trust also have information on volunteering opportunities.

11. Still life photography

Still life photography can be used as a mindful meditation by looking. It is taking the time to really explore what you are seeing.

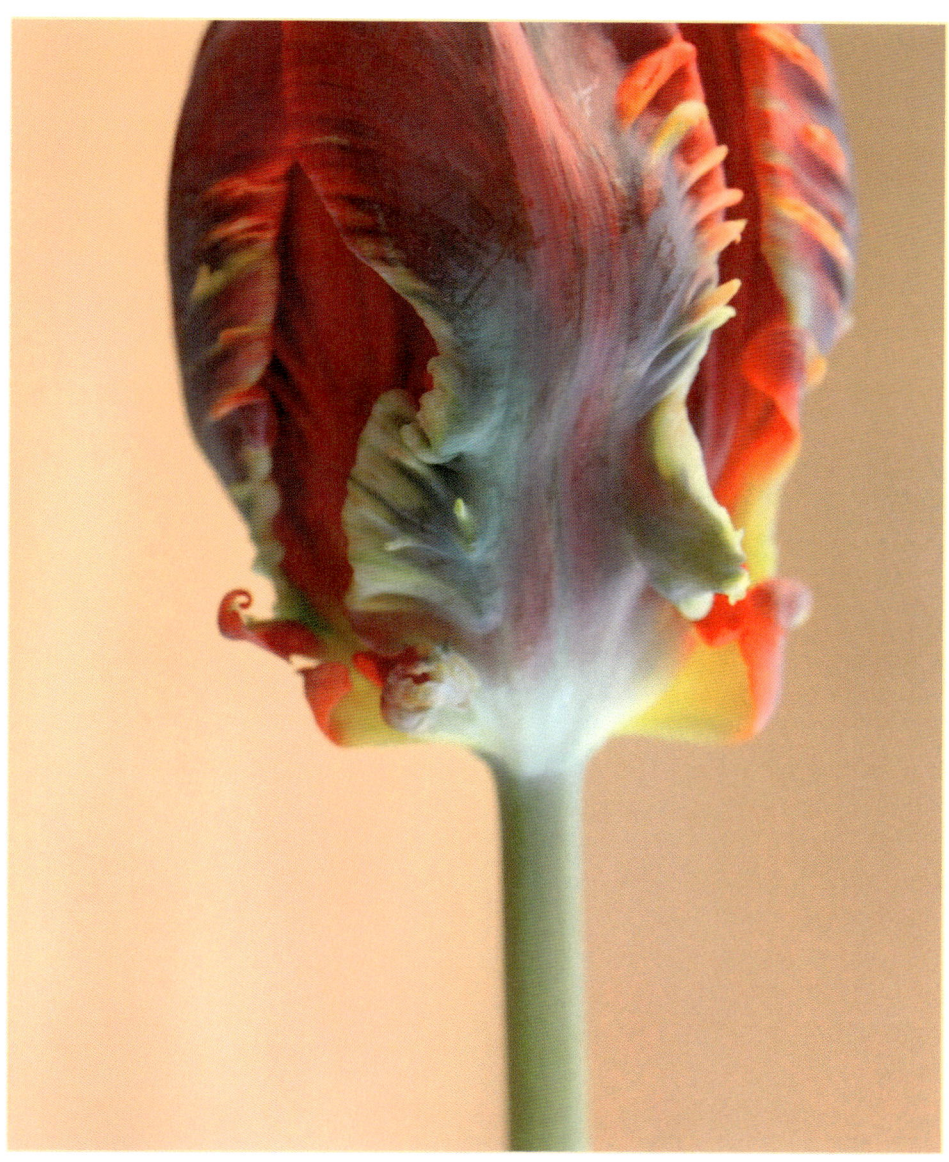

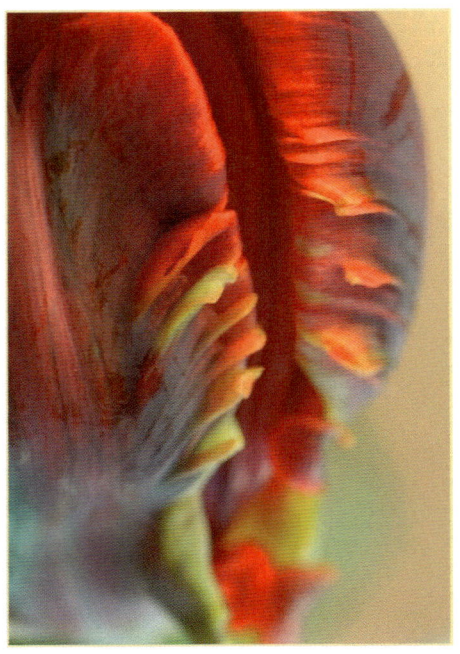

This project is based around mindfulness and nature, but there are still ideas on how to make it more social and creative below. Choose something to photograph, it doesn't have to be of a natural object but it's a good way to connect with nature if you choose one and can reveal beautiful detail that you may not have noticed. Try and capture the shapes and colours, how the light falls on the object. Here I have chosen tulips; my favourite flowers but you could go on a mindful walk and pick a bunch of wild flowers. When I started to look at the tulips I hadn't noticed the blue until I really looked or the layers of colours. Taking photographs from different angles revealed more details on the petals.

Make it more social

You could find and enrol on photography course. I did a short course at night school to learn how to use my SLR camera and basics of taking a good photograph. Use this link to find further education courses in your area https://nationalcareersservice.direct.gov.uk/course-directory/home (there may be a cost for courses).

The photographs above I had printed as greetings cards to give to people.

Make it more creative

Experiment with different exposures angles and filters. Try different light sources.

Try lino cuts of your photographs by transferring the outline onto lino using graphite paper.

Write a Haiku about what you are seeing (see Chapter 7, Write).

Print your photos to make a collage, cut out words that come to mind when you see the images and stick them on, make it a collage for your wall or decorate a table top (remember to seal it), box or book cover.

Take it forward

The International Garden Photographer of the Year (IGPOTY) is an annual competition that people can enter at a cost, but also has a gallery of photographs to inspire you

https://igpoty.com/.

Wildlife Photographer of the Year is an annual competition run by the National History Museum that anyone can enter for a fee http://www.nhm.ac.uk/visit/wpy.html but the website has a gallery of photographs to inspire you.

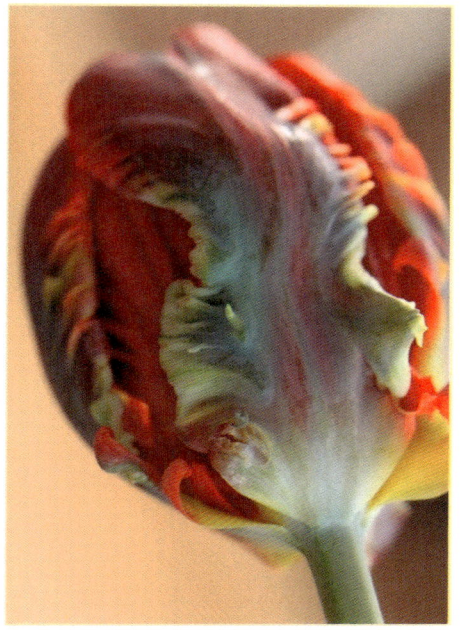

III. Your favourite place

This project involves going to your favourite place with your phone or camera and capturing the beauty of it to make images that remind you of that place at other, perhaps more stressful times. I use them as screen savers at work.

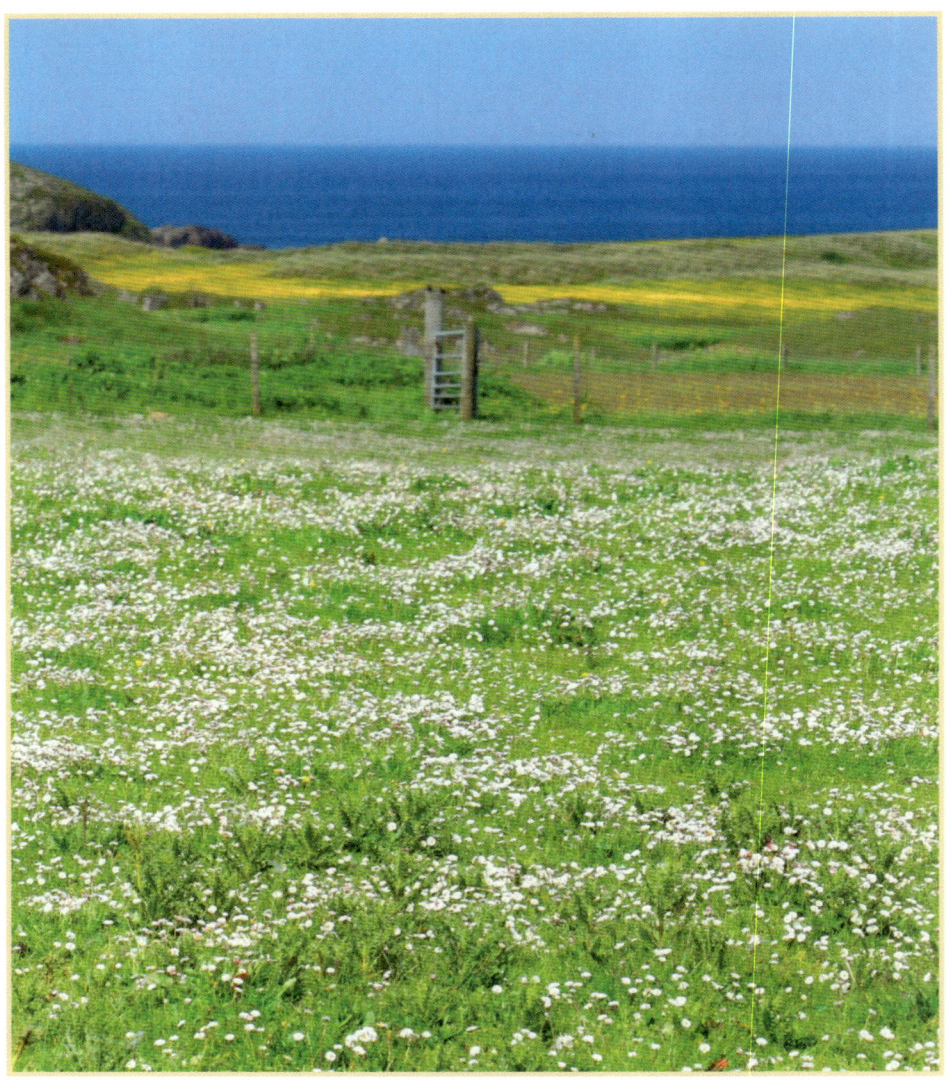

This project is based around mindfulness, creativity and nature, but there are still ideas on how to make it more social and an exercise in mindful looking that can be done indoors following on from this project below.

Try and choose somewhere that you feel calm and peaceful. Try and photograph it on a day when the light is good and take photos of different parts, perhaps a journey through it or the details you see as you walk. Be creative in your approach to capturing what really makes this place special for you. You could take a short video on your phone to capture the sounds and movement around you, or a 360° perspective to make you feel like you are actually there afterwards.

Although you don't have to choose somewhere in a natural environment as some people prefer architecture or cityscapes, research has shown that just looking at a picture of the natural environment can evoke similar health benefits to actually being there, so this project might be one that you can try to see if it works for you. The mindful looking exercise below can be done with any photo, painting, drawing, sculpture or just the view from your window.

Make it more social

Join a walking group or photography group.

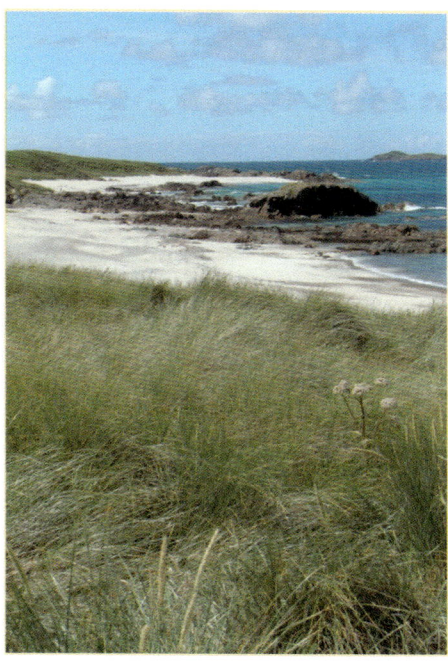

Go on a walk with a friend and take a picnic, perhaps with the summer salad in Chapter 4, Cook.

These photographs are from a holiday I took in Scotland, on the Isle of Mull and Iona. When I travel alone I tend to stay in youth hostels, which keeps the cost down but is also a very social way to travel. Follow this link to find out more about the Youth Hostel Association, but there are many good independent hostels too www.yha.org.uk.

Make it more mindful

Breath deeply and slow your thoughts, spend time just sitting first and immersing in what you can see, hear, smell and touch then begin to take your photographs

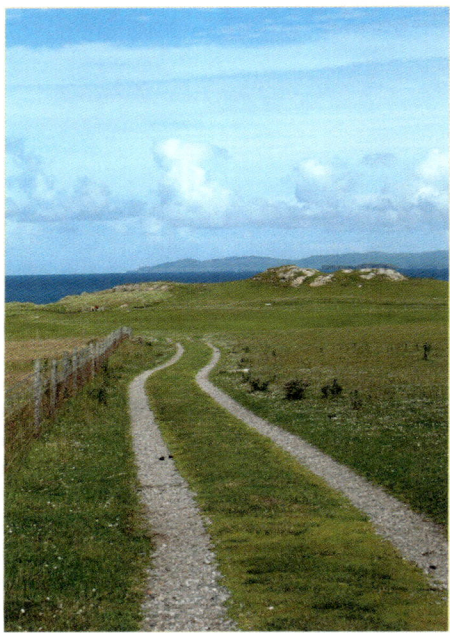

Use the photographs as a looking mindful meditation. This involves scanning the image slowly with your eyes, working your way through it from the top left hand corner to the bottom right hand corner, noticing the shapes, forms, colours, details and any feelings it evokes. Notice any distracting thoughts as you do this and gently let them go.

For example, in the photograph above:

Follow the shoreline with your eyes.

How many shades of blue can you see?

What can you see on the horizon?

What do you notice in the foreground?

Is the sea calm?

How many different types of plants can you see?

How many different shades of green can you see?

Take it forward

Schedule in your next visit to your favourite place.

Plan in holidays or days out to find your next new favourite place.

CHAPTER 4

Cook

"The table is a meeting place, a gathering ground, the source of sustenance and nourishment, festivity, safety, and satisfaction. A person cooking is a person giving. Even the simplest food is a gift."

– Laurie Colwin

I. Autumn roasted vegetable soup

This is a warming thick soup, full of flavour. It's a versatile recipe for any time of the year, just use whatever vegetables are seasonal.

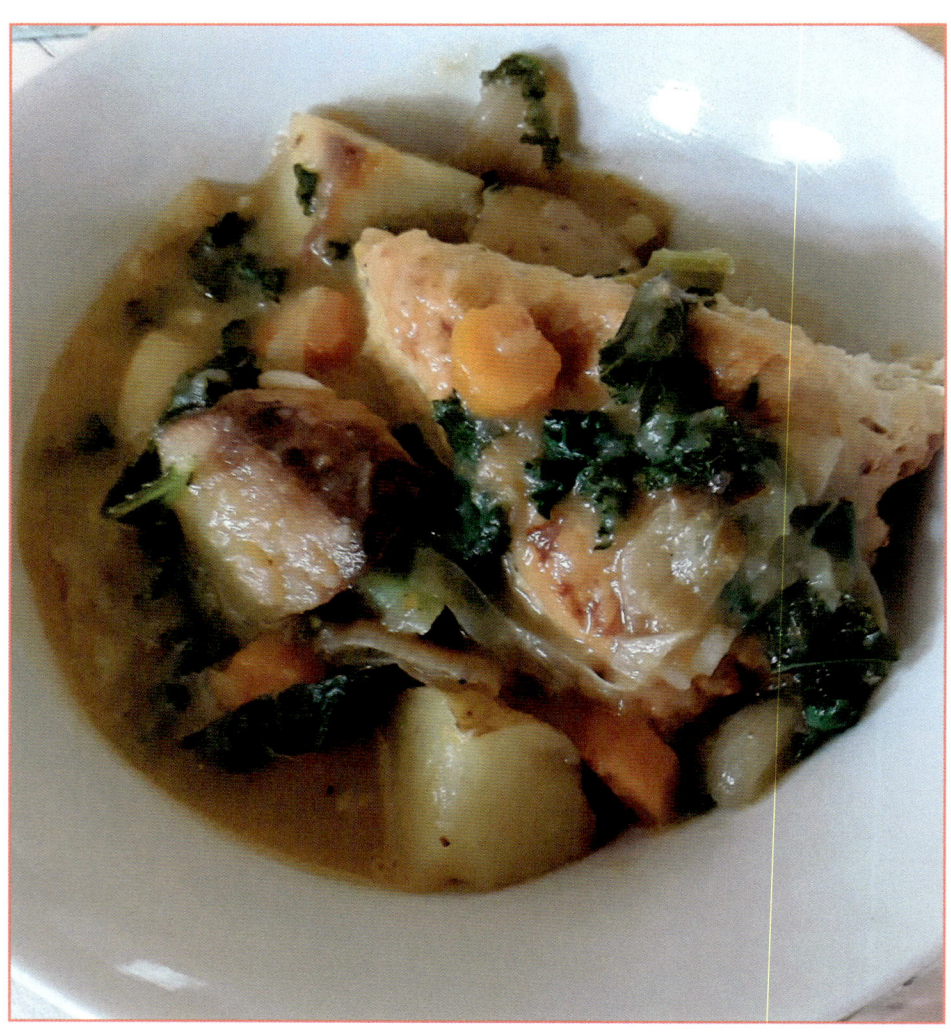

Ingredients you will need:

(makes enough for 4 people)

- 3 medium sized leeks, trimmed, with the outer layer removed and thinly sliced.
- 1 tbs of olive oil, plus extra for drizzling
- 4 medium potatoes cut into chunks, leave the skins on for extra taste.
- 5 medium carrots peeled, trimmed and cut into chunks.
- 6 shallots trimmed, peeled and cut into quarters.
- A large handful of chopped curly kale with the woody stems removed.
- 6-8 sprigs of fresh thyme.
- 1 bulb of garlic broken into cloves but unpeeled.
- 2 pints of good quality vegetable stock.

Equipment you will need:

- Vegetable peeler
- Knife
- Chopping board
- Large deep baking tray
- Large saucepan
- Wooden spoon
- Electric hand blender (these can be purchased for under £10 in electrical stores or supermarkets)
- Measuring jug

Method

- Preheat the oven to 200°C (fan 180°C, gas mark 6).
- Prepare the leeks, carrots, shallots and potatoes and put them in a large bowl with a tablespoonful of olive oil and toss them until they are coated.
- Spread them on the deep baking tray.
- Put the garlic cloves and sprigs of thyme on top of the vegetables and drizzle over a little more oil.

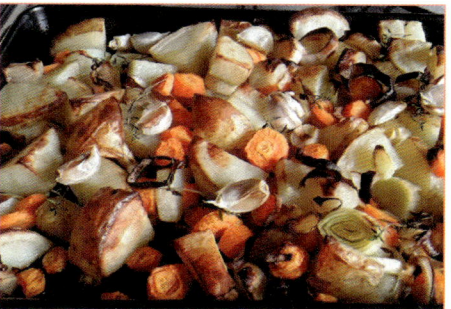

- Roast for 45 minutes until the vegetables are soft and slightly charred.
- Discard the thyme and squeeze the garlic out of the cloves over the vegetables.
- Put half of the vegetables in the large saucepan with the 2 pints of vegetable stock and blend with a hand blender.
- Put the kale on top of the other half of the vegetables and return to the oven for 5 minutes.
- Tip the kale and vegetables in with the stock mixture and heat gently.

- Season to taste.
- Enjoy on its own or poured over a cheese and herb scone (see Chapter 1, Bake).

Add your favourite recipe combination to your journal and take photographs of your meal, add tips and ideas for the next recipe.

Make it more social

Invite friends for lunch and try preparing the recipe together.

If you work, start a lunchtime soup group in your workplace as it's a good way to get to know people better and make time to enjoy your food.

If you are going to a party, offer to prepare this recipe to share.

Make it more mindful

If you are using home grown vegetables, spend time choosing what you are going to pick. Notice the different colours of the ingredients and the different smells as you chop them. Taste the vegetables and herbs as you cook. Notice the smell from the oven as the vegetables roast and the smell of the soup gently heating. Notice the taste of the soup and the texture in your mouth.

Connect with nature

Grow the vegetables and herbs to cook with (see Chapter 2, Grow).

Take the soup in a flask as a warming lunch on a walk.

On a bright sunny autumnal day, if you have any outside space, wrap up in warm clothing and eat al fresco.

Take it forward

https://www.bbcgoodfood.com/ has lots of free recipes for cooking and baking.

The OneYou phone app is free and has healthy quick and easy recipes with the option to add ingredients for your chosen meal automatically onto a shopping list, ideal if you have a busy schedule.

Make it more creative

Be curious and adapt the recipe to your taste. Try different vegetables, herbs and flavourings. Learn to make some fresh artisan bread to eat with it.

11. Summer salad

This is an easy colourful salad with sweet and savoury flavours. The edible flowers add interest and colour to the dish as well as providing subtle flavours that you can be mindful when tasting.

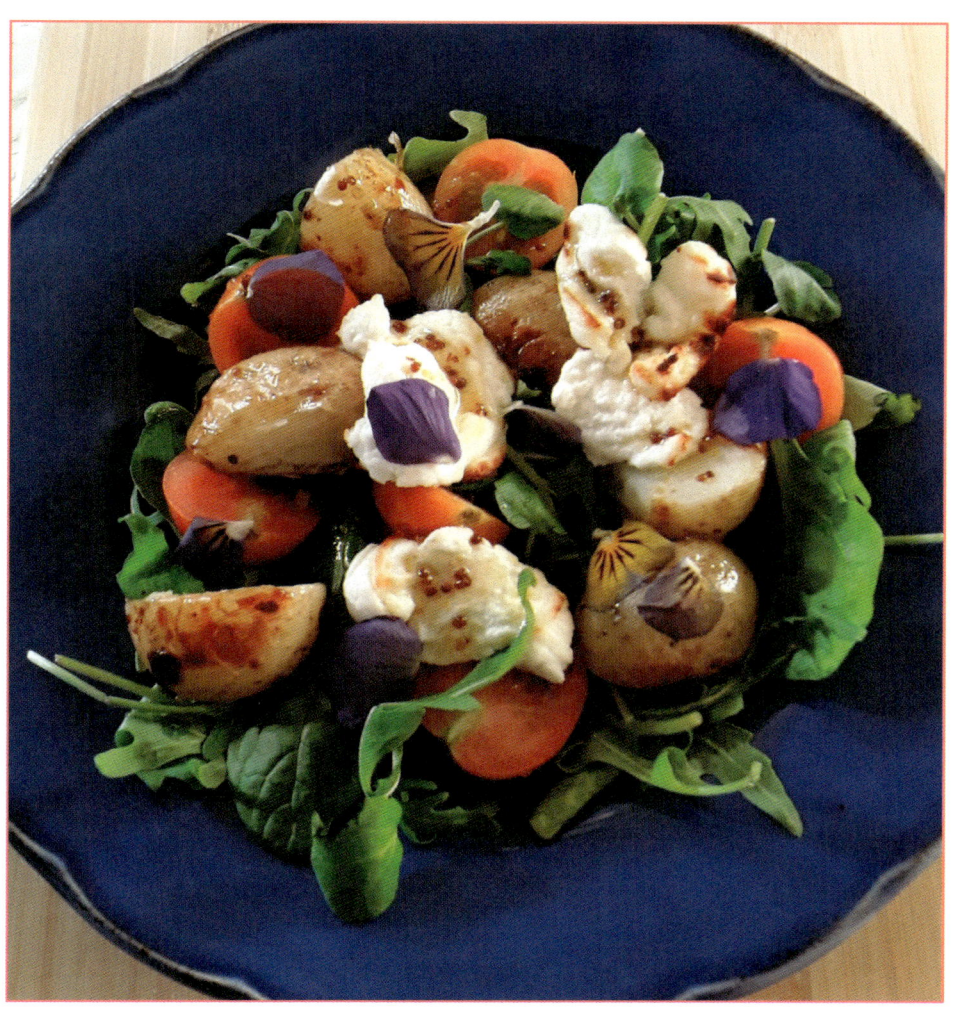

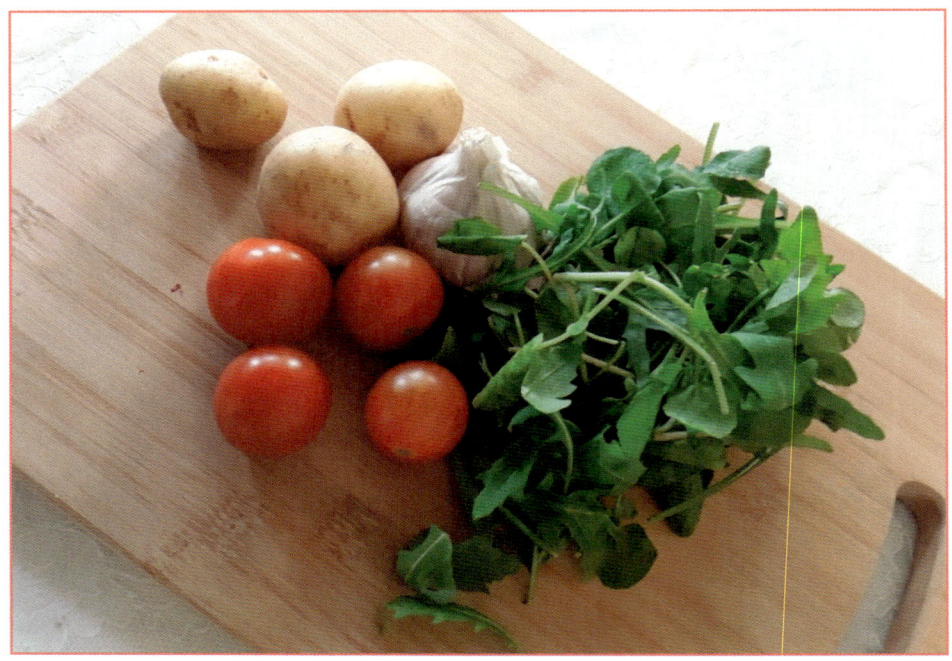

Ingredients you will need:

(serves 1)

- 50g goats cheese log cut
  into 1cm thick slices.
- A good hand full of rocket,
  watercress, and spinach
- 5 cherry tomatoes cut in half
- 6 new potatoes
- Runny honey
- 5 gloves of garlic
- A small bunch of edible
  flowers such as pansies, picked
  fresh and rinsed well.

For the dressing:

- 1 tbs of olive oil
- 1 tsp honey
- ½ tsp wholegrain mustard

Equipment you will need:

- Chopping board
- Knife
- Saucepan
- Small dish
- Baking tray
- Strainer

Method

- Preheat the oven to 200°C
  (180°C fan or gas mark 6).

- Put the potatoes into boiling
  water in the saucepan and
  simmer for ten minutes, then
  strain them, put them on a
  roasting tray, drizzle with honey
  and olive oil and add 5 cloves of
  garlic. Roast for ten minutes.

- Wash the salad leaves and place in a bowl.

- Cut the tomatoes in half and arrange on top of the salad.

- When the potatoes are done (soft in the middle and golden brown on the outside) arrange them on top of the salad.

- Put the cheese slices on a baking tray and grill for 1-2 minutes on a medium heat until it starts to melt and turn brown. When it's done, put the cheese on top of the salad.

- Mix the olive oil, honey and mustard in a small bowl and drizzle over the top.

- Garnish with the edible flowers and enjoy.

Make it more social

Double the ingredients and share it with a friend.

Make as a side dish to take to a party to share.

Post a photo on social media.

Connect with nature

Try growing your own vegetables, edible flowers and herbs (see Chapter 2, Grow)

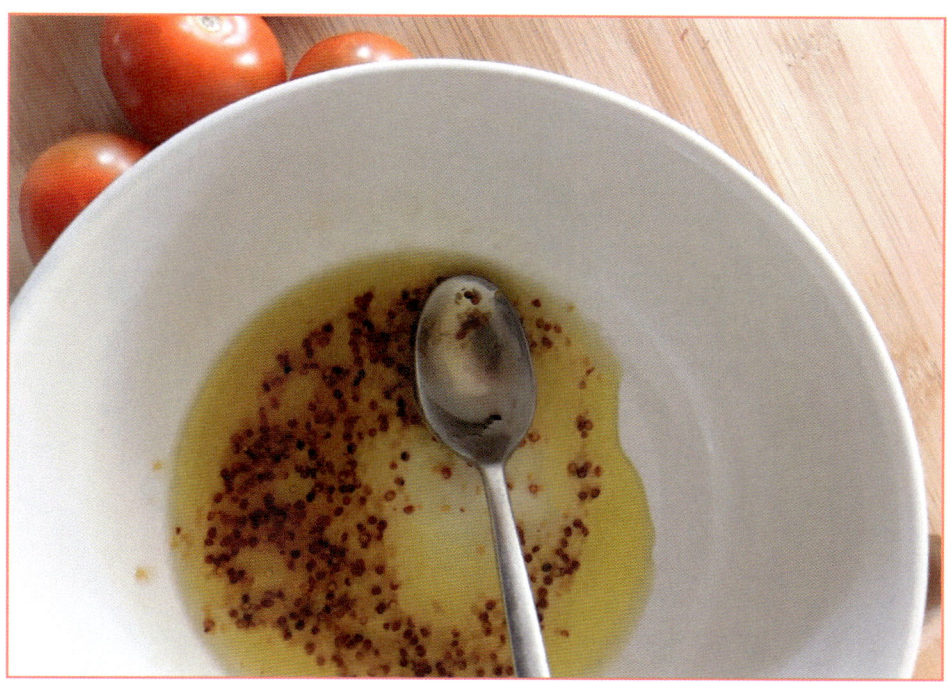

Find a local foraging course and go along to meet other people and reduce the cost by using wild ingredients. Make sure you always know what you are picking as some plants are poisonous.

Make it more creative

Experiment with different ingredients, flavours, textures, and edible flowers to make the salad to your taste.

Add your favourite combination to your journal and take photographs of your meal, add tips and ideas for the next recipe.

Experiment with different salad dressings.

Bake some artisan bread to have with your salad.

Make it more mindful

If you are using home grown vegetables, spend time choosing what you are going to pick. Notice the different colours of the ingredients and the different smells as you chop them. Taste the salad, flowers and herbs as you cook.

Notice the different textures of the ingredients in your mouth and the sweetness of the honey, sharpness of the cheese and heat of the mustard seeds.

Take it forward.

Find other recipes that use edible flowers.

Visit charity shops for recipe books.

Find a cookery course in your area.

Watch some cookery programmes for inspiration.

Schedule in your next cooking day.

III. Christmas chutney

This chutney goes really well with cheese and has Christmassy flavours as it uses ginger and nutmeg, but the recipe can be easily adapted for other times of the year.

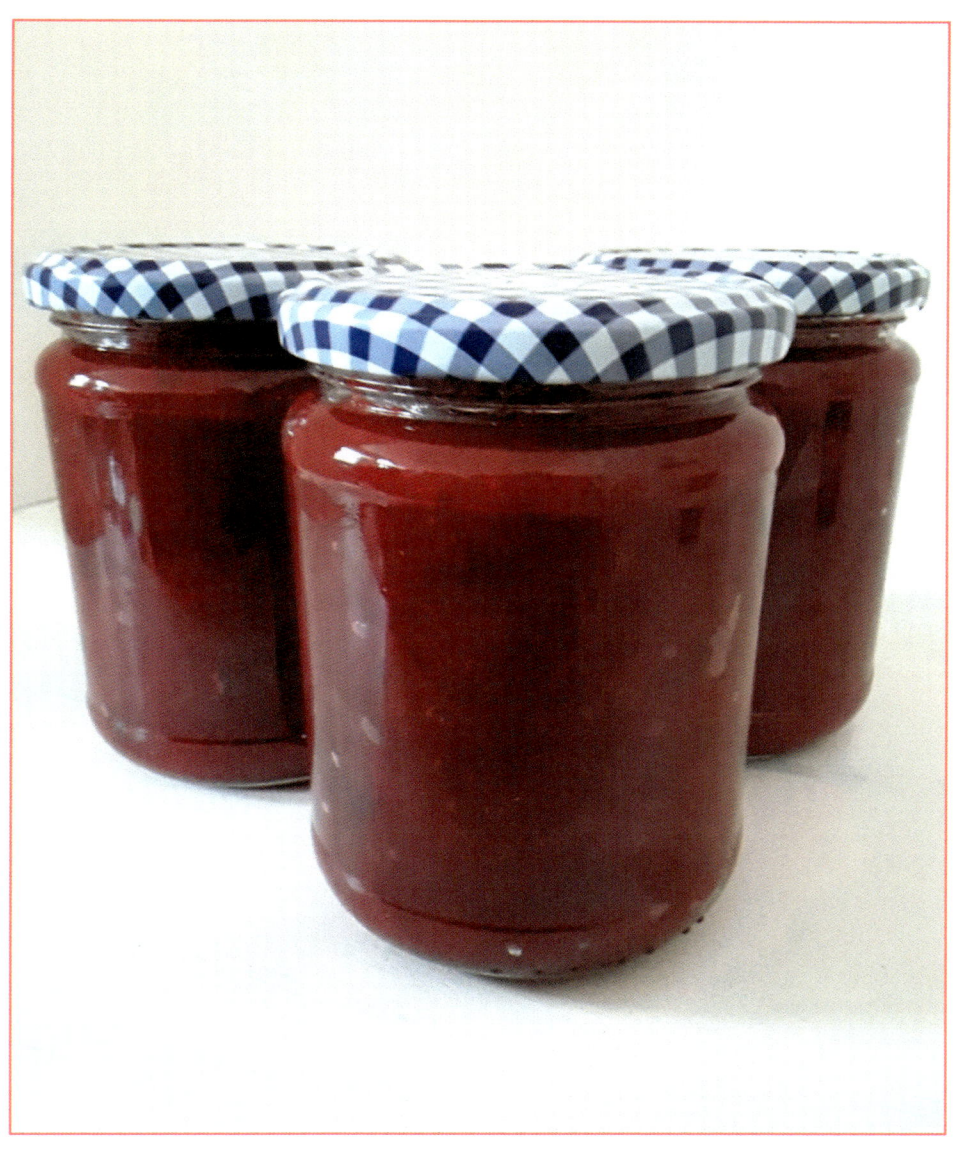

Ingredient you will need (makes four 300ml jars):

- 1 ½ lb (pounds) beetroot peeled and chopped into 1cm pieces (wear gloves to do this as the juice will stain your hands).
- 1lb apples, peeled, cored and chopped into 1cm pieces.
- 1Ib red onions finely chopped
- 1Ib red cabbage, thinly sliced
- The zest and juice of 2 oranges
- 400g of soft brown sugar
- 350mls white vinegar with a malt percentage of 5% or above
- 1 tsp ground ginger
- 1 ½ tsp grated nutmeg
- A splash of vegetable oil for cooking the onions

Equipment you will need:

- Four 300ml jam jars
- Rubber gloves
- Knife
- Chopping board
- Peeler
- Large saucepan
- Baking tray

Method

- Cook the onions over a gentle heat in a little vegetable oil until they are translucent and softened. Add the vinegar and sugar and heat until the sugar has melted. Add the beetroot, apple, ginger, orange juice and zest, and simmer and reduce until the apples have fallen and the consistency is of a thick paste (this can take up to 60 minutes).

- Preheat the oven to 160°C (140°C fan, gas mark 3).

- Wash the jars and lids thoroughly by hand in warm soapy water, rinse, drain but don't dry them and put them on a baking tray in a hot oven for 10-15 minutes to sterilise them.

- Pour the chutney into the jam jars whilst the chutney and the jars are still hot and seal them. Leave for the taste to develop for at least a month.

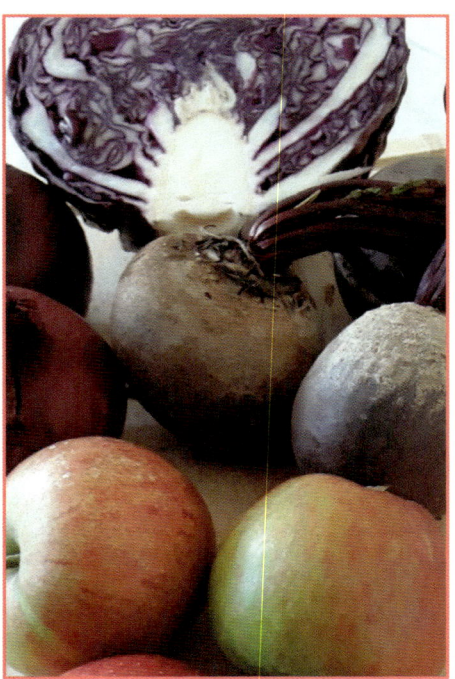

Make it more social

This chutney makes an ideal Christmas gift. Add a square of cloth over the lid, secure with an elastic band and add a label.

Pack the chutney and some cheese and herb scones (see Chapter 1, Bake) to share on a walk or to have a picnic with friends.

Connect with nature

Grow your own vegetables and fruit (see Chapter 2, Grow).

After you've been on a foraging course, try recipes with wild produce like hedgerow crops.

Make your own paper with pressed flower petals for the labels on your jars.

Make it more creative

Add your recipe to your journal, again with ideas to try for the future, photographs and illustrations.

Try different recipes and flavourings, be creative and curious. Why not try a spiced chutney with chilli. Try using

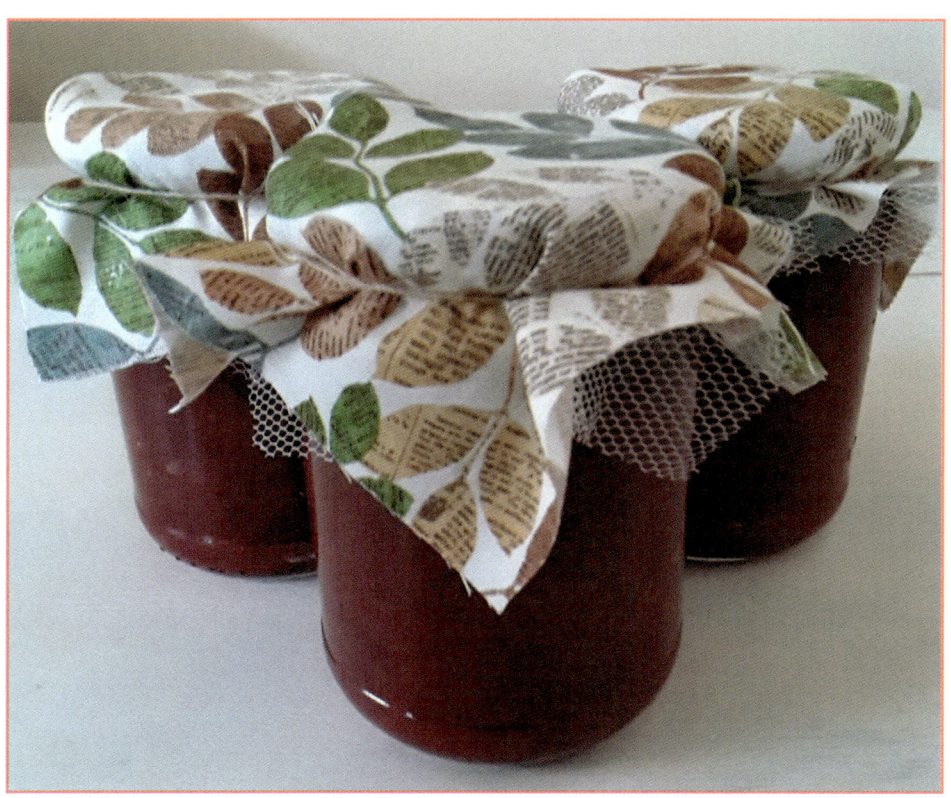

ingredients that that you haven't tried before.

Draw illustrations on your labels.

Make it more mindful

Slow down.

If you are picking your own ingredients, take your time to choose which to use.

Smell the orange as you zest it, taste the ingredients, notice the different colours, notice the smell of it cooking and if it changes as it cooks.

When you taste the chutney, take your time to find the different flavours and try it with different cheeses and breads or scones.

Take it forward

If you grow your own vegetables, plan in your next chutney making day by looking at the harvesting calendar.

Look for jam and other preserve recipes and try those too.

Look for workshops on preserving produce near you.

Visit farm shops on your walks to get some inspiration on new recipes.

CHAPTER 5

Craft

"Make gifts meaningful by putting the time in creating them, whether baking and cooking, or in making arts and crafts. It will all have more meaning for the giver and receiver."

– Lidia Bastianich

I. Leaf necklace

This project captures the forms of nature in detail and can be adapted to match your favourite colours. It can also be made into a keychain by attaching it to the hook from a pound token.

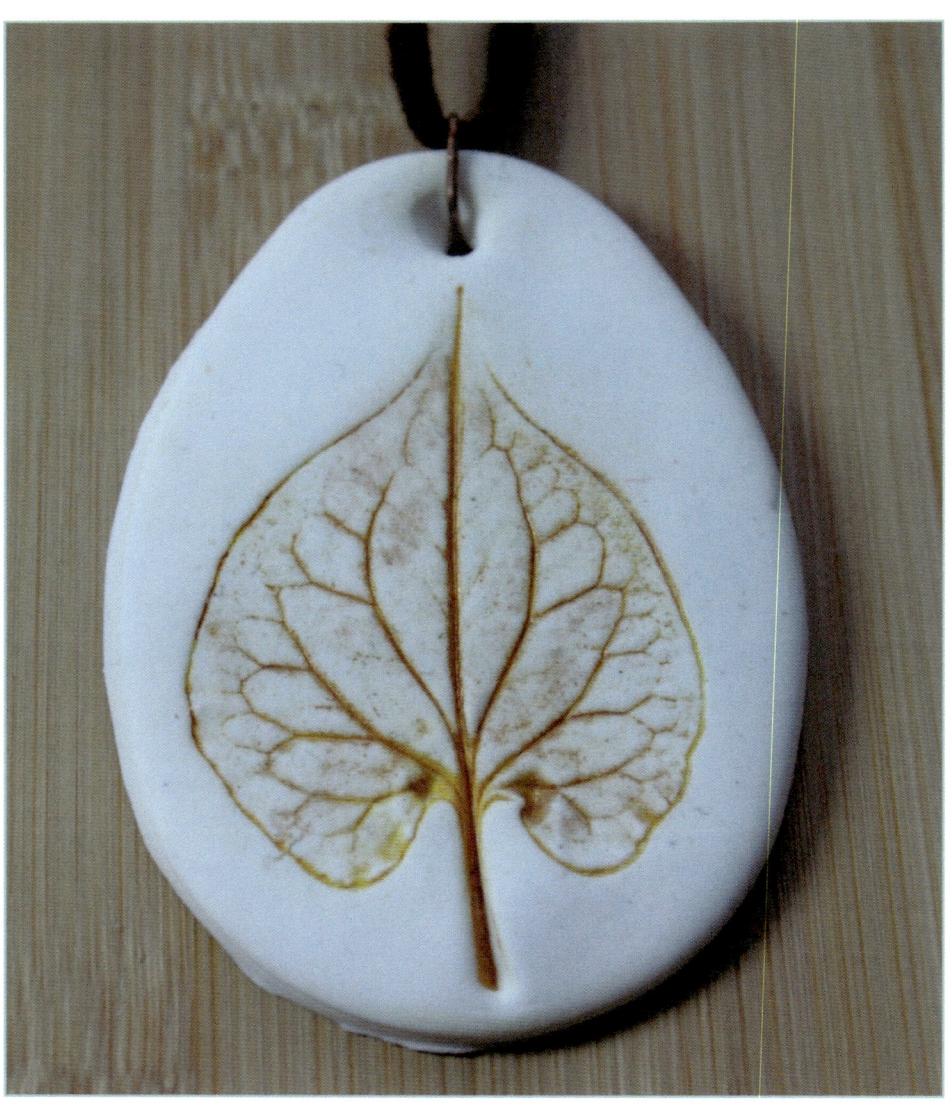

Materials you will need:

- 2oz soft polymer clay, oven hardening, in the colour of your choice
- Rolling pin
- Greaseproof paper
- Biscuit cutter, I used 6cm oval shape
- Collection of natural objects, leaves, flowers, seeds, feathers, whatever you like as long as it's flat
- Metal jewellery ring to attach the pendant to your chain
- Chain
- Large needle or toothpick to make the hole at the top
- Acrylic paints and paint brush
- Nail varnish remover and cotton buds

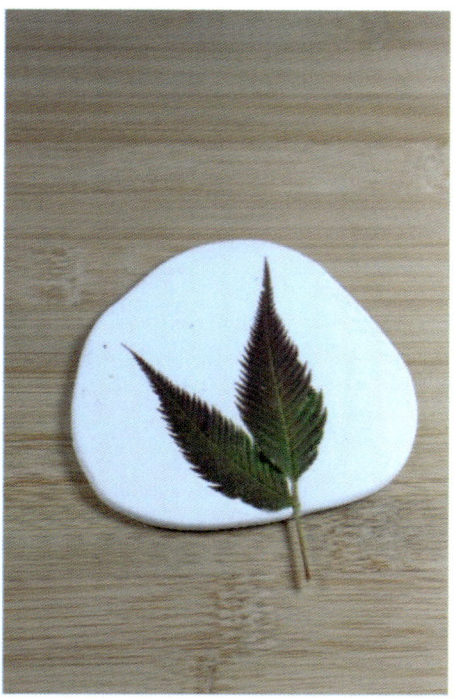

Method

- Work the clay in your hands for a couple of minutes until it is soft and pliable.
- Divide the clay into 4 equal pieces and work with one at a time.
- Use the rolling pin to roll out the clay on the greaseproof paper until is it approximately ¼ inch thick.
- Gently press your chosen natural object onto the clay, position in the centre or off centre.
- Turn the clay over and gently roll the back with the rolling pin.
- Turn the clay over again and gently lift the object.

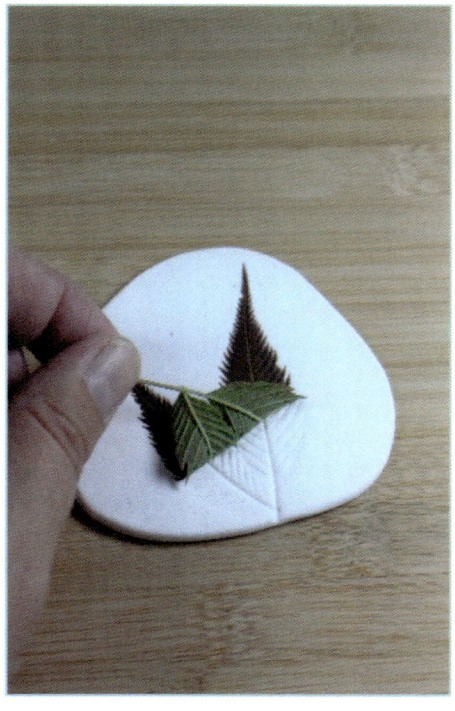

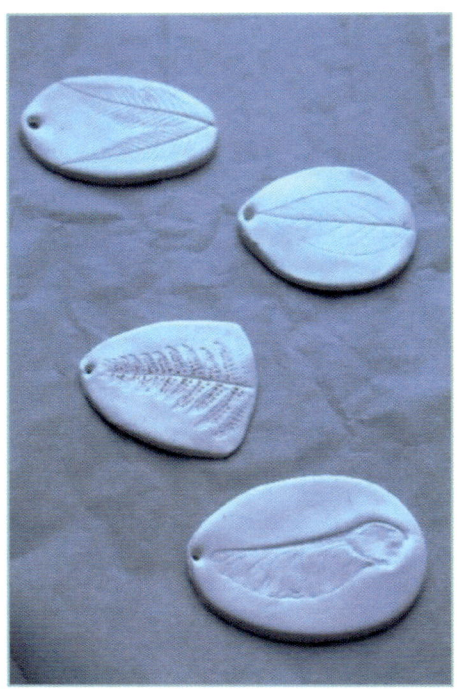

- Cut the clay to size with your biscuit cutter, or shape it yourself.
- Poke the needle or toothpick through the top to make a hole.
- Complete for all four pieces of clay.
- Follow the baking instructions on your clay, but mine was baked at 130°C fan for 30 minutes.
- Remove from the oven and allow to cool
- Paint over the entire surface of the clay with acrylic paint, and then wipe off gently with the nail varnish remover on a cotton bud to take off all the paint except that caught in the details. Reapply as necessary.
- Attach to a necklace with the jewellery ring.

Make it more social

Find and enrol on local craft courses to learn new skills and meet people with similar interests.

Make a piece for someone you know that's personal to them in some way,

Make the pendant from a natural object collected on a group walk.

Connect with nature

Gather objects on a mindful photography walk (see Chapter 3, Photograph).

Photograph the most interesting natural objects before you press them into the clay (see Chapter 3, Photograph).

Wear your very own piece of nature.

Make it more creative

Use metallic paints and glitter to highlight areas of your design.

Use the pieces in a mosaic (see the project below).

Make different sized pieces to be used as coasters, or ornaments to be hung from a tree in the garden or at Christmas.

Make it more mindful

As you collect your natural objects, look for interesting shapes and feel the textures.

Notice the detail in the print.

Notice the detail that is highlighted as you add paint.

Take it forward

Schedule in your next crafting day.

Research other crafts you might like to try on the internet.

Look for local jewellery making courses and enrol on one.

Visit http://www.creativecrafts-online.co.uk/ the Creative Crafts Association website of craft fairs in the North West of England that you can visit for inspiration and materials.

II. Autumn colour inspired textile piece

It's lovely to spend time outside on a fair weather day, but by doing this project you'll also have a lovely textile piece to take home with you.

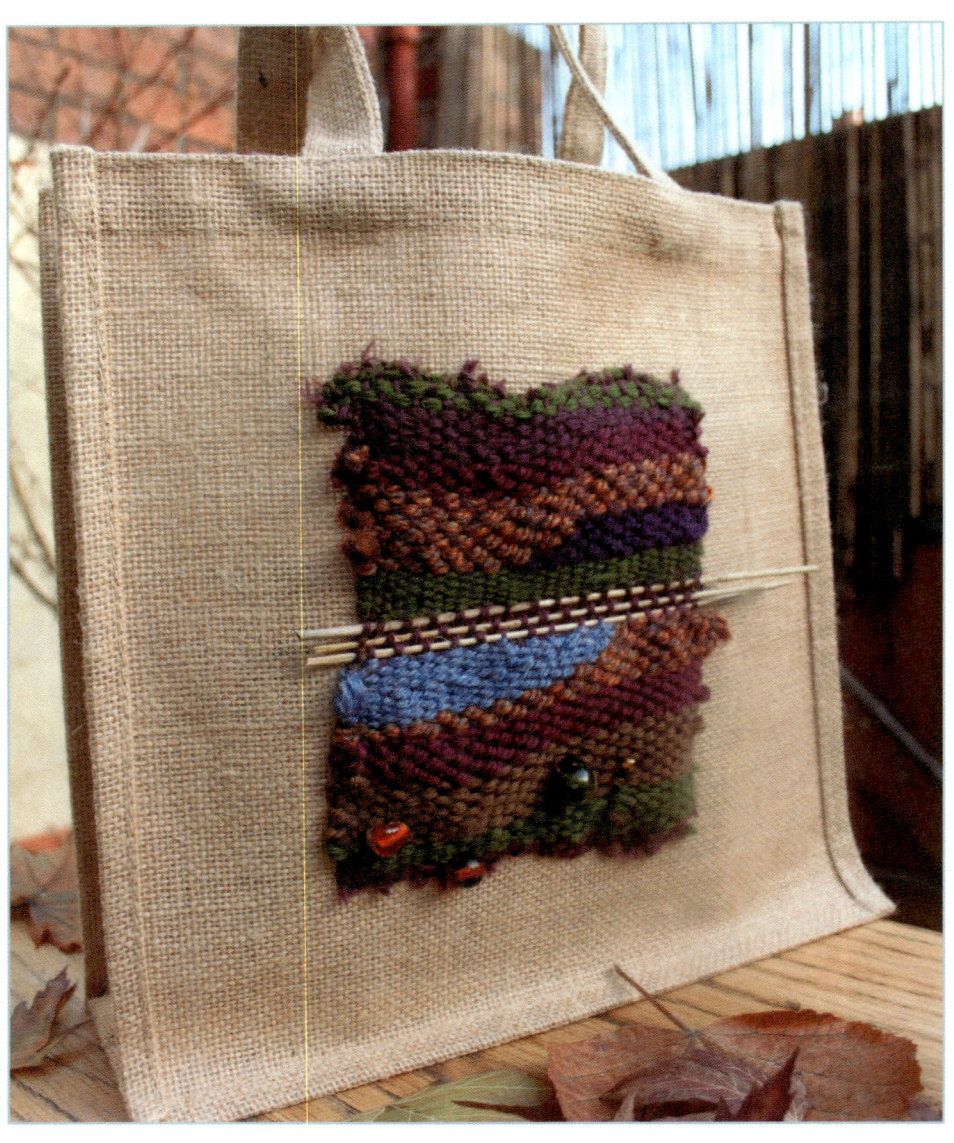

Take different coloured threads and material, yarn, whatever textile mediums you would like to use and find a comfortable space to sit outdoors in a place you find beautiful.

Embroider, weave or knit a small piece inspired by what you see.

This is a piece I began weaving one October in the Lake District. I was inspired by the leaves beginning to turn golden, reds, oranges, yellows and the purples of the heather, browns of the bracken and green ferns on the fells contrasting with the blue water. I used wool and tapestry yarn with glass beads and wove in grass from my walks with my dog Eric.

Make it more social

Make the piece into a greetings card, bag or book cover for a friend.

Embroider a larger piece inspired by the one produced today onto a table cloth, handkerchief or cushion as a gift.

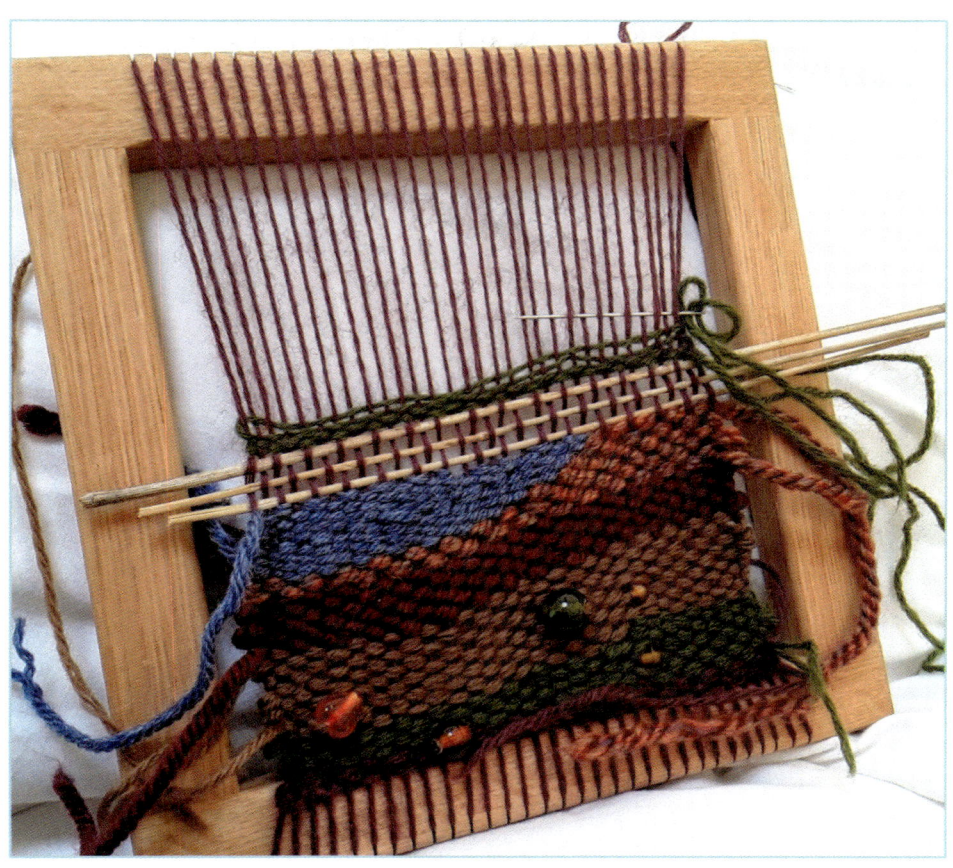

Knit a scarf or blanket based on the colours of your piece as a gift or to sell.

Shop locally in independent shops for your materials and speak to staff for advice.

Join a "Knit and Natter" group, these are usually free and can be a source of help and feedback on your work.

Connect with nature

Autumn is a truly breathtaking demonstration of what nature can do with colour, but every season has its own beauty. Try doing this project at different times of the year and notice how the colour pallet changes.

Make it more creative

Collect interesting items to incorporate into your design or make a frame with twigs or weave them into your piece.

Be inspired by the space as a whole and try and capture some of the colours and/or shapes with your piece, or concentrate on one detail.

Look for any patterns such as fractals or natural mandalas and use these for inspiration.

Make it more mindful

When you go for a walk, spend some time just noticing what is around you, what you can see, hear, smell, touch. Be aware of being in this place, in this moment. Notice the light and the colours around you. Look for details but also for impressions of the environment as a whole. Feel the textures of the yarns, beads, threads and objects you have collected. Make them fit together in the right way to represent where you are at this moment.

Alternatively, embroider on natural objects, and make a collage or cards.

Take it forward

Find and book onto a related course such as crochet or knitting.

Check Meetup for textile related groups in your area, register and sign up.

Start your own group. See the concept of Hugge or Croodle for ideas on cosy winter groups.

Learn to colour your own yarns with naturally produced dye extracted from roots and plants (see Chapter 6, Make art).

III. Beach walk memory mosaic

This project incorporates a walk on a beach, mind-fully looking for "treasures" to take home and create something beautiful to remind you of the day.

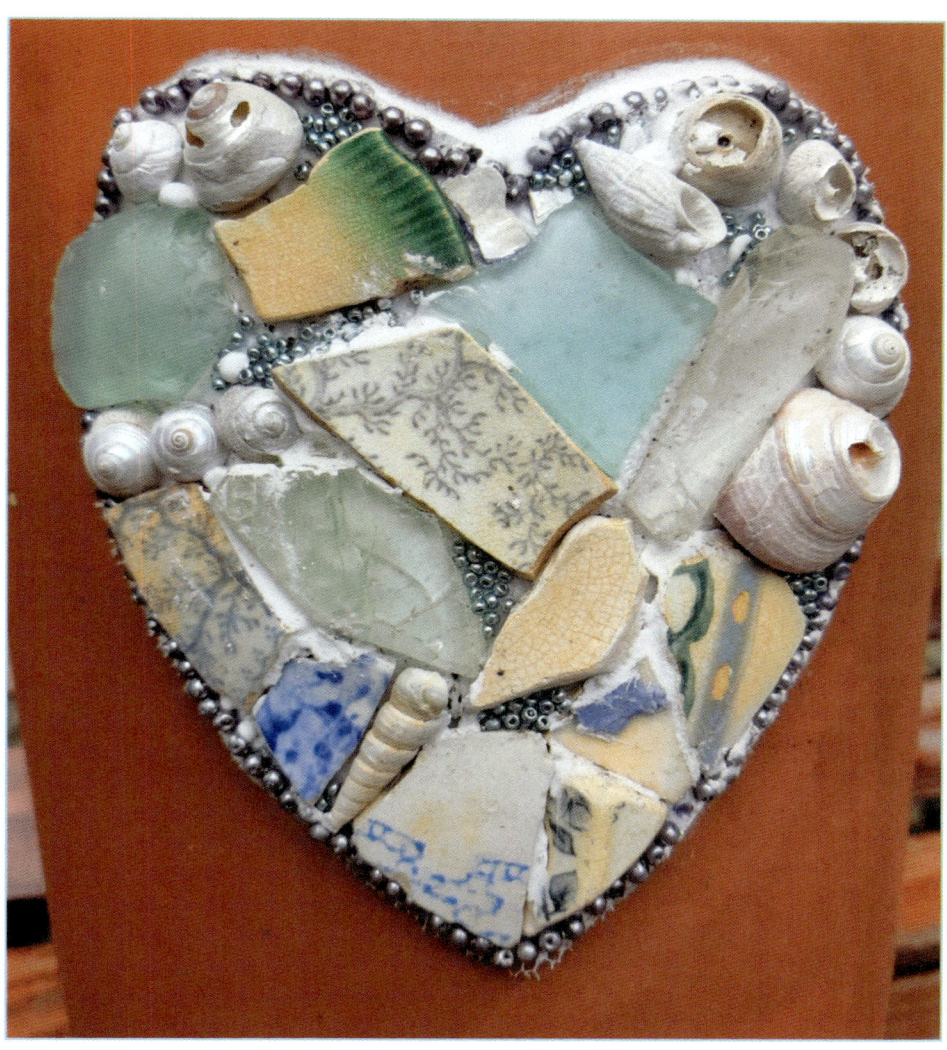

Decide on a location or locations to visit. I did my mosaic with gathered items from my holiday, so I collected them over a week. You are looking for shells, sea glass, and old pieces of pottery that you can build your mosaic with (being careful not to take away anything that is a home for something, such as hermit crabs or disturb the natural environment too much).

When you have gathered your objects, decide on the size of the mosaic and what you are going to do it on. I decided to use a terracotta plant pot for my garden.

Materials you will need:

- A piece of Tulle fine mesh fabric
- A pencil
- Tile grout
- A pallet knife
- Fine grain sand paper
- Cling film
- Old newspaper
- Rubber gloves
- A pair of scissors
- A good selection of natural objects
- An old cloth

You can also gather other items to add into your mosaic, I added beads to form the heart shape and fill in the gaps.

With the pencil draw the outline of the shape you want your mosaic to be onto the Tulle and lay it onto a piece of cling film. Put the Tulle and cling film onto

newspaper if you are using a kitchen work top. Put on your gloves.

With the pallet knife, gently add a layer of tile grout about a centimetre think within the shape, and make sure you go right to the edges.

I then pressed a string of beads into the grout to make the outline of the shape, and then pressed in the objects. When you are happy with your design, leave it to dry for at least 12 hours.

When fully dry, cut around your shape and gently rub the back with sandpaper to remove the cling film. Apply a thin layer of grout to the back of your design and position it onto the plant pot. Smooth around the edges with your finger and wipe off any excess with an old wet cloth. Leave to dry and enjoy your memories preserved in the mosaic.

Make it more social

Find and enrol on a mosaic making course.

Make gifts for people with personalised mosaics.

Organise your trip to the beach with a friend (visit Crosby beach to experience Another Place by Antony Gormley www.anthonygormley.com to see how nature is reclaiming the beach).

Connect with nature

Try and identify any wildlife you see on your walk. What birds can you see and hear? What lives in the rock pools if there are any on the beach? What kind of plants are growing in this environment? Carefully lift rocks to find out what's there and put them back gently. Identify wildlife with a book or the internet.

Make it more creative

Sketch some of the items in your journal.

Make a natural mandala with your found items and photograph it before you collect them up and leave.

Mosaics can be any shape so try and make one that represents the place where your items were found.

Try adding mirrored tesserae, marbles or glitter to the tile grout to reflect the light.

Make it more mindful

Spend time on the beach noticing the colour of the sea and sand, the sound of the waves, the bird calls, the different shapes of your gathered objects, the smell of the air and seaweed. Take off your shoes and feel the sand under your feet, paddle in the water.

Take it forward

Schedule in your next visit to the beach.

Look for inspiration in other pieces of mosaic on the internet, or research other forms.

CHAPTER 6

Make art

*"Every child is an artist. The problem is how
to remain an artist once we grow up"*
– Pablo Picasso

I. Autumn leaf printing

This project involves using the beauty of natural objects to make art and is a great activity to do with your children.

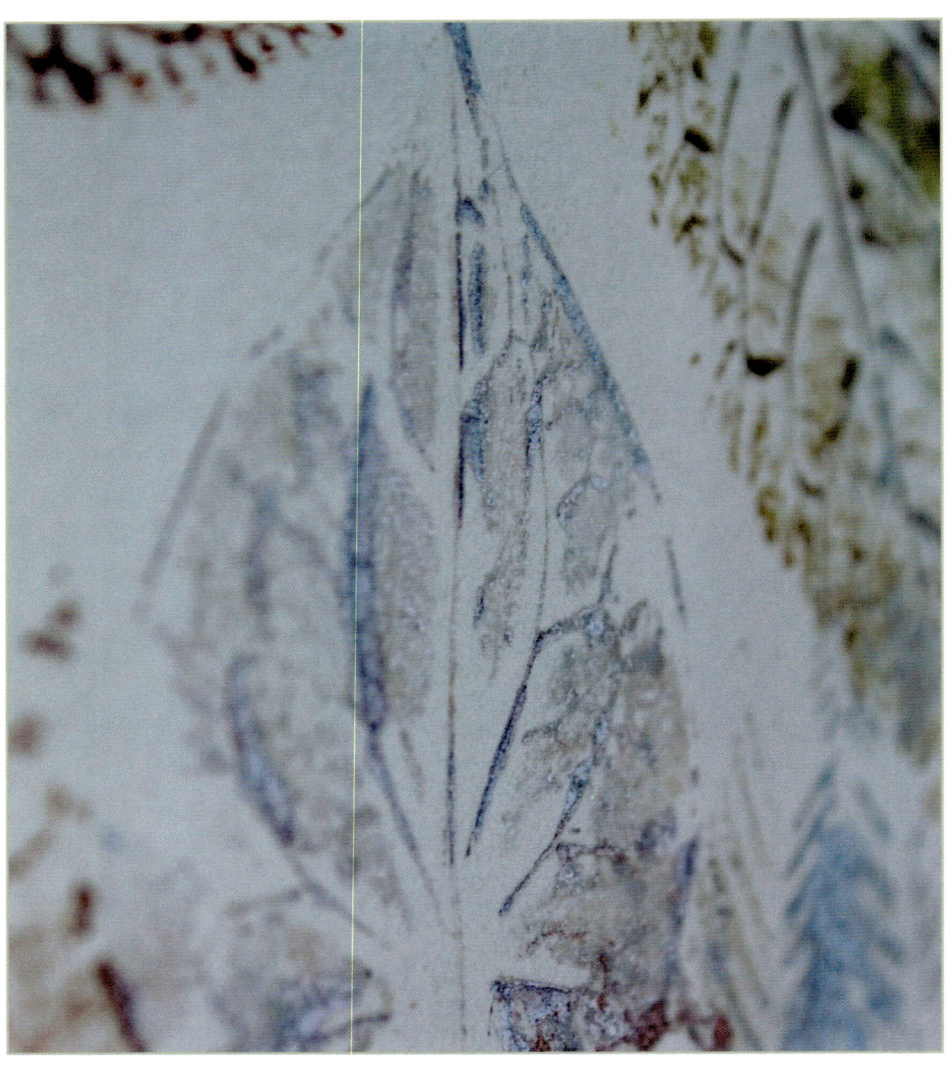

Materials:

- Old newspaper to cover your worktop
- Acrylic paints of your favourite colours
- An old saucer to mix the paint on
- A paint brush
- Pieces of watercolour paper
- Some natural objects such as, leaves, seeds, and flowers, feathers, whatever you like as long as it's flat, has some texture and is clean and dry.

Method

- Choose a natural object and lay it flat on the covered worktop. Pour small amounts of your paints onto the saucer and chose a colour. Some objects such as leaves may have a side that has more texture than the other so choosing this side will give the most detail to your print. Dab the paintbrush into the paint and apply it to the side of your object that has the most texture, making sure to go right to the edges.
- Press the object gently onto the paper; lift off straight up being careful not to smudge the paint as you remove it.
- Alternatively try a heat pressed print. You will need to gather some leaves around autumn time. Try and collect the ones with the brightest colours. Coat both sides

of one leaf with white vinegar with a small paintbrush and sandwich it between two sheets of watercolour paper. With a hot steam iron, press down on the paper for 10 seconds at a time, being careful not to scorch it and moving the iron all over the paper for approximately one minute. Very carefully turn the sandwich over and repeat on the other side. Allow to cool, then lift off the top sheet and carefully remove the leaf to see the imprint. Your leaf is also now dried and preserved.

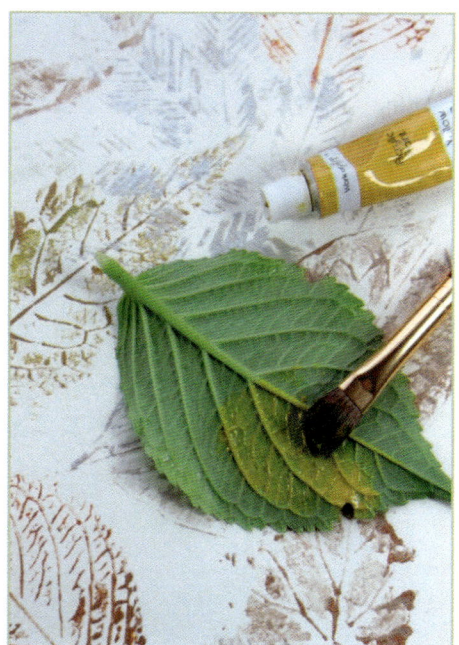

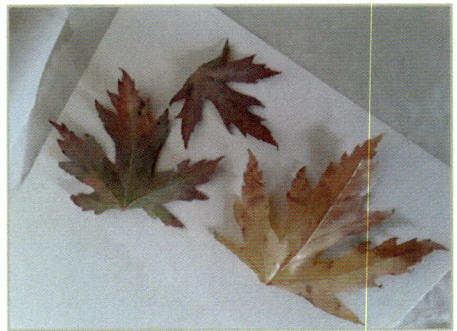

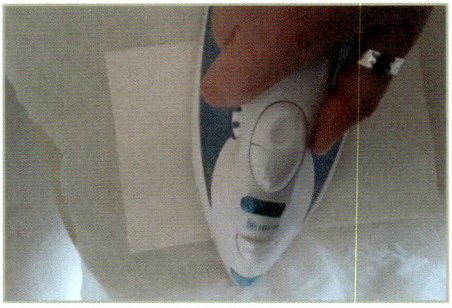

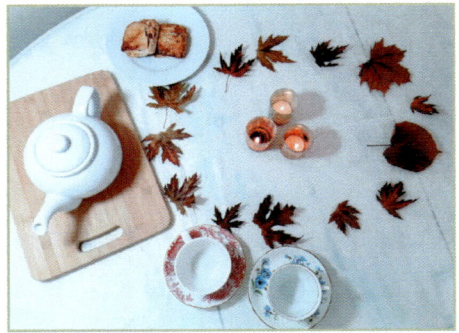

Connect with nature

Go on a nature walk to collect your natural objects. Spend time searching for different shapes and textures. Be inspired by the colours in nature around you when choosing your colours. If it isn't raining, do this activity outside and print objects as you go.

Make it more creative

Make a collage of different coloured prints. Try using metallic coloured paints, glitter paints or sprinkling glitter onto the wet paints. Make your own paper, adding dried crushed leaves or flower petals to complement or contrast with the colours of paint you are using. Paint or draw designs around the leaf print.

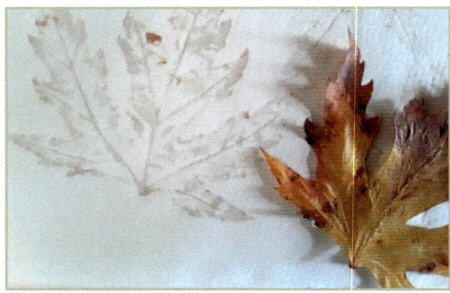

Make it more social

Stick your prints onto blank greetings cards for any occasion. Try to choose shapes, colours or designs that a particular person will like. Make a card or picture with objects collected on a nice day spent with someone else to remind you of it.

Use the dried leaves to decorate your dining table when friends visit for tea.

Make it more mindful

Notice the shapes of the objects, feel the texture of them, try mixing different colours of paints to find the ones you like. Notice the pressure as you make the painted prints. Do the paints have a smell? Feel the glitter between your fingers as you lightly accent your work. If you are working with others, notice their responses to the activity.

Take it forward

Look at other artists who draw inspiration from the natural world, Claude Monet, Vincent Van Gogh and Paul Cezanne are some of my favourites but also look for lesser known artists in local art galleries, they might have regular free talks or events that you can get involved with.

https://www.royalacademy.org.uk/exhibitions-and-events the Royal Academy in London, England is open to the public and has exhibitions and courses, some free and some at a cost.

The Tate gallery has a website with lots of different artists work and a section on special exhibitions and art activities for children which can be just as much fun for adults www.tate.org.uk.

Schedule in your next art session, perhaps to produce Christmas cards or a project for someone's birthday.

11. Mandala

The mandala (translated as "circle") is a Tibetan Buddhist visual aid for concentration and meditation. You don't need to follow the Buddhist faith to make a mandala, but ideas from other faiths and cultures can add to our toolbox of occupations that we find therapeutic.

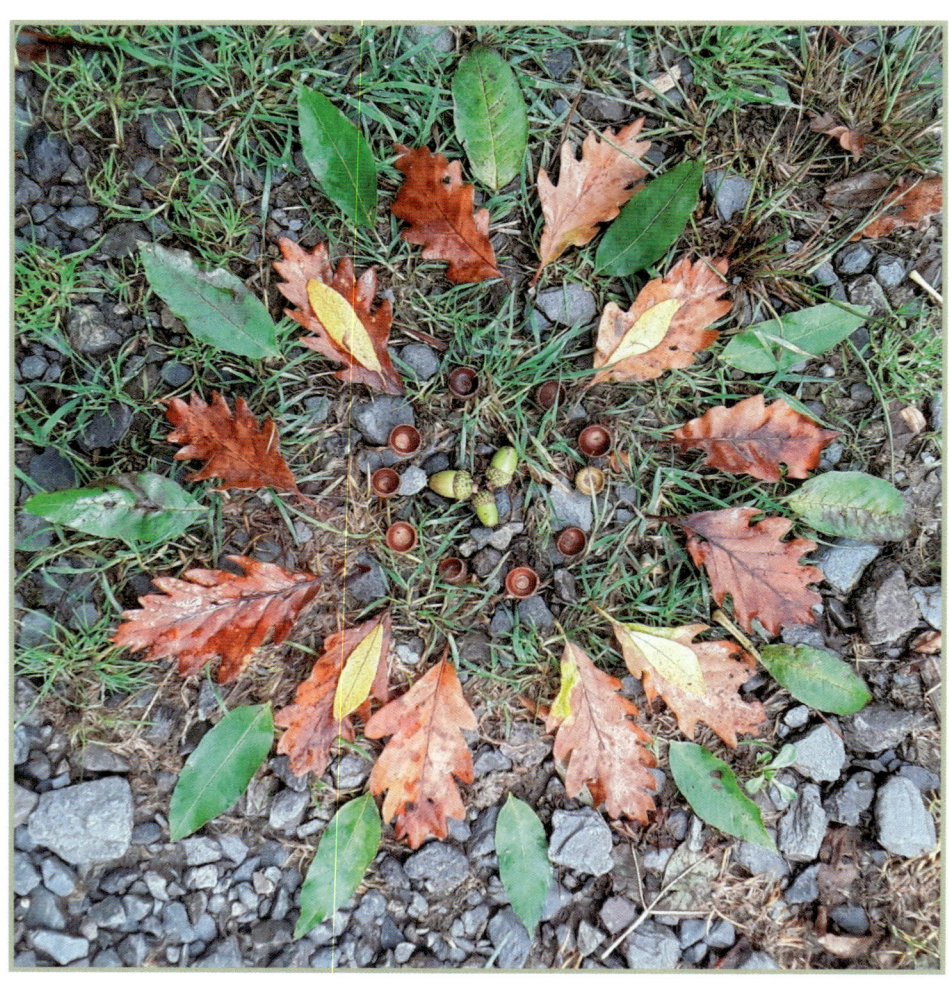

In this project you will be making your own mandala and experimenting with different mediums. Your instinct about the design and colours should guide you through the process of creating your own. There is no right and wrong way to do it as it is a form of self expression, but the pattern tends to be repeated in the traditional form as this can help us to focus. Carolyn Mehlomakulu is an art therapist and psychotherapist who suggests that drawing a mandala can be therapeutic as it promotes centering, meditation, emotional expression and is self soothing. Personally I find draw-ing a mandala a calming and mindful activity (see http://creativityintherapy. com/2012/11/mandalas/)

You could start by drawing on paper before making your natural mandalas.

Method

- https://www.art-is-fun.com/ how-to-draw-a-mandala This website has a great step by step guide to drawing a mandala.
- This is how I draw a mandala:
- You will need a square piece of paper, a compass, a pencil, a ruler and some different coloured pens or pencils.
- Use a ruler to draw two straight lines from corner to corner, crossing in the middle of your page.
- Place the end of the compass on the center of this cross

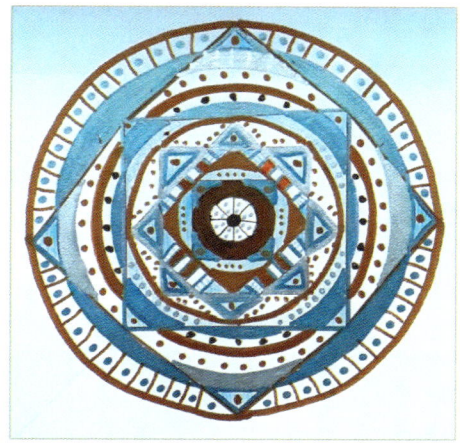

and draw a small circle in the center of your page.
- Keeping your compass in place but opening it out in stages, draw larger circles radiating out from the center circle, as many and as spaced out as you want.
- Start making shapes and patterns on your mandala using colours but make it repetitive, so if you draw a shape in one circle, draw it again to make a pattern in that circle.

- To make your natural mandala, see the beautiful work of James Brunt for inspiration on his website http://www. jamesbruntartist.co.uk/mandalas/.
- The natural mandala will be a temporary piece of art that will return to nature over time, so remember to take a photograph or draw it when you have finished.
- Go to a natural space like a beach or park and find a quiet space that is not on a main path

- and is relatively flat and large enough for your mandala.
- Gently clear the area of stones or fallen leaves or flatten your chosen area of sand.
- Explore the area around your space for objects to make your mandala. Remember you are looking for a repeating pattern so if you choose leaves then they should be of a similar shape, size and colour.
- Place an object in the centre of the space then work outwards adding patterns to your mandala until it feels complete.

Make it more social

http://www.Mandalaproject.org/About/Index.html

The project founded by Lori Bailey Cunningham is a worldwide project that aims to bring people together to create something larger than themselves and celebrates unity and diversity via the symbol. The website has lots of resources, so why not set up a group to make a quilt mandala.

Connect with nature

The circle with a center pattern is recurrent in nature, flowers with petals radiating from the center, the concentric rings of a tree, and the spiral of a shell, why not go for a walk and see how many

you can find to draw or photograph for inspiration? When you are preparing fresh fruit and vegetables, look for mandala's in the form and structure.

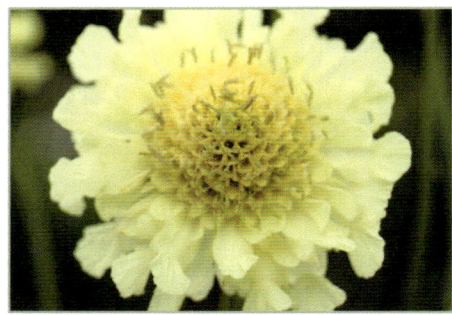

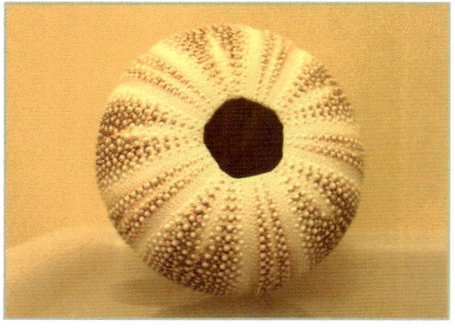

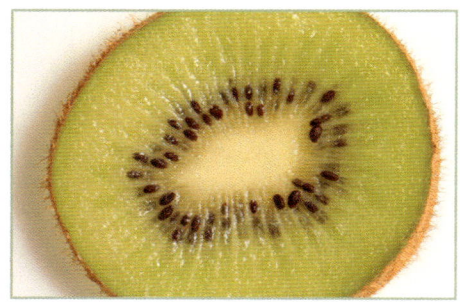

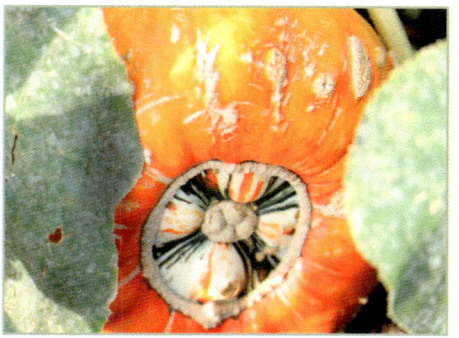

Make it more creative

Use beads, sequins, repeated designs from wrapping paper, shapes cut from old book pages etc to stick on to your drawn mandala.

Make a cross stitch mandala.

Make an appliqué design with material and use it as a wall hanging or cushion cover.

Make it more mindful

When you are out on a walk, search for shells, pebbles, leaves, seed heads, flowers to press, feathers etc to stick onto your design in your journal. These will need to be of similar shape and colour to repeat your pattern.

Take it forward

Schedule in your next art session, or keep your journal with you and try mindful doodling.

Research mandala's on the internet to understand more about how they can be used to meditate.

Find a local meditation class to explore other ways of doing this.

Find a local art class to see if other types of painting has the same meditative affect.

III. Easter eggs

This project is fun to do at Easter, but can be done any time of the year to make unique and colourful ornaments. The use of natural dyes is creative and can give unusual and unpredictable results.

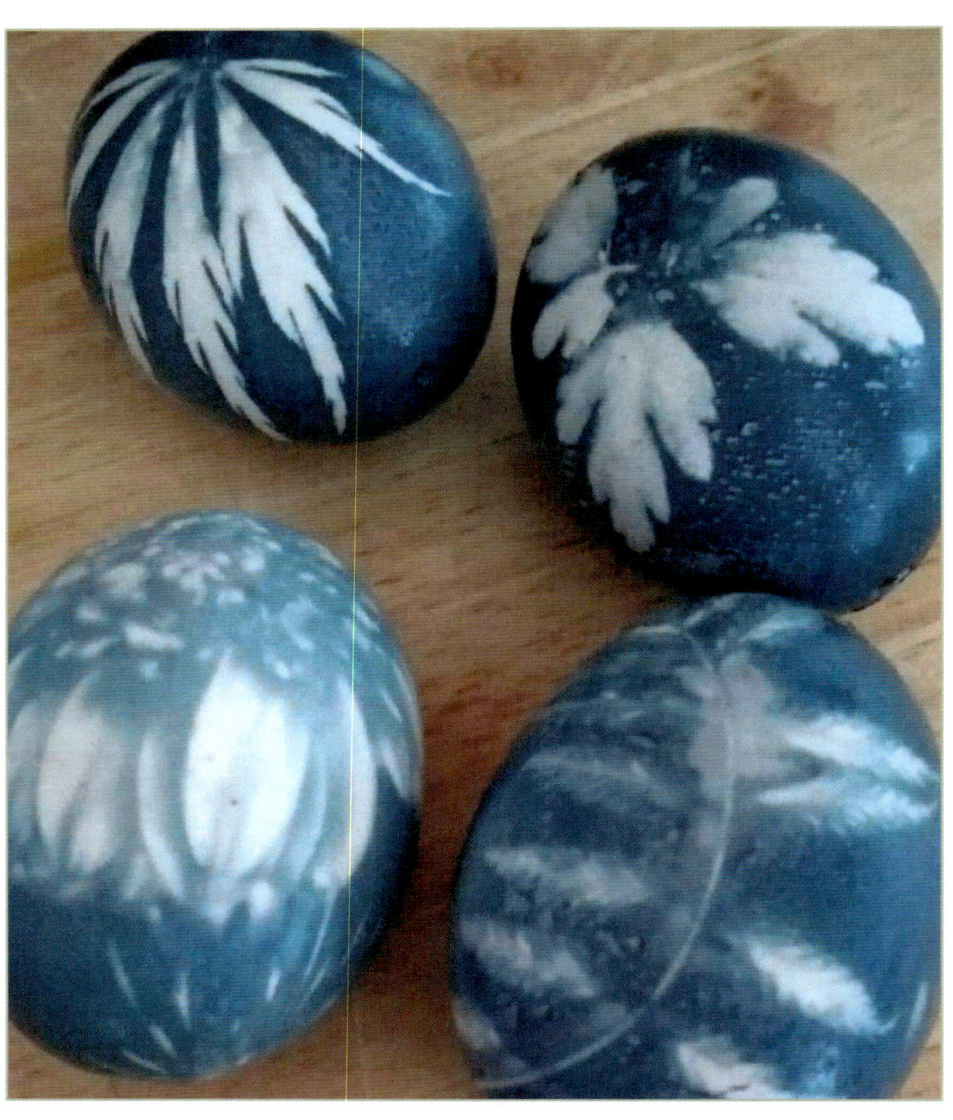

Materials:

- Half a red cabbage
- Knife
- Chopping board
- 4 eggs (white if possible but brown ones will turn green)
- A large saucepan
- Vinegar
- An old stocking or pair of tights
- An elastic band
- Fresh flowers or leaves
- A large jug

Method

- Shred the cabbage into small pieces with the knife and place it in the saucepan with enough water to cover it by 1 inch.
- Bring to the boil and simmer for 40 minutes.
- Strain and discard the cabbage, allow the liquid to cool, and then pour it into the jug with 1 tablespoonful of vinegar.
- The eggs can be hard boiled or blown but I find the blown ones last longer. To blow an egg, pierce two small holes in the top and bottom of the eggshell with a sharp thick sewing needle then blow into one hole to force the yolk out of the other one.
- Choose a flower or leaf and place it onto one of the eggs, securing with a taught piece of material from the tights or stockings and an elastic band. Repeat for the other 3 eggs.

- Place all the eggs in the dye and fully submerge them by placing something that will not stain on top, like a small dish or large cup.
- Leave for at least 12 hours in the fridge.
- Remove from the dye and remove the elastic band and material, then peel off the flower or leaf.
- Rinse gently under a cold tap and rub them gently with your fingers to remove any excess dye, leave to dry.

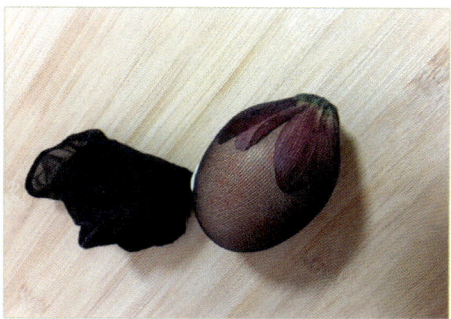

Make it more social

These eggs make great gifts for people and if blown will last for a few months. Carefully gluing string around the egg will make it into a hanging ornament.

This project is great done with friends, perhaps with a nice home cooked lunch (see Chapter 1, Bake and Chapter 4, Cook).

Connect with nature

Grow your own flowers and vegetables to make the natural dyes.

Go on a walk and forage for interesting leaves and flowers.

Make it more creative

Experiment with other natural dyes: turmeric, onion skin, tea etc.

Tie die fabrics with your natural dyes.

Add burnishing to the design using metallic paints and try painting instead of dyeing with a stipple effect to give a realistic speckled egg pattern.

Glue on beads, buttons, yarns, words from the newspaper or magazines.

Make it more mindful

Focus on colours and designs. Try detailed work such as a mandala design with paints (see above).

Notice the patterns in nature that you are transferring onto the egg.

Take it forward

Schedule in your next art session.

Find and enrol on an art course.

Visit art galleries.

Find out more about natural dyes and their uses. Try dying yarn to make your nature inspired textiles.

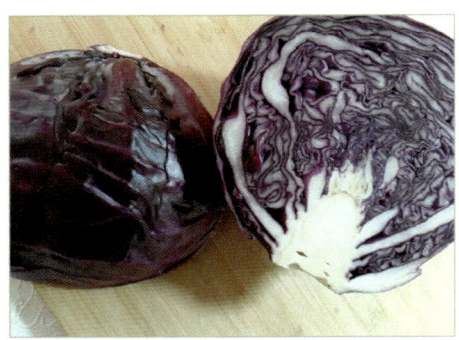

CHAPTER 7

Write

"Writing means sharing. It's part of the human condition to want to share things-thoughts, ideas, opinions."
— Paulo Coelho

I. Nature journaling

The following project involves using writing as a medium to help us to connect with nature and be more mindful but there are also suggestions to help you make it more social and creative.

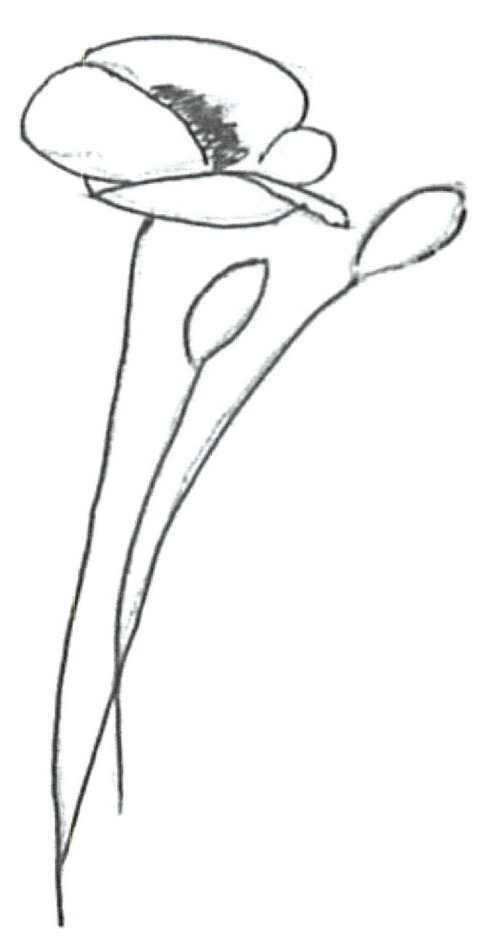

Take your journal out with you when you head to a natural space e.g. garden, park, woodland, allotment etc.

Spend some time just noticing what is around you, what you can see, hear, smell, touch.

Do any or all of the following:

- Make notes about the season and any changes you are noticing.
- Use a bird, insect or plant identifier and name what you can see and hear.
- Write about how what you are seeing makes you feel.
- Write down any questions you have about what you are seeing.

Make it more social

Visit your local community charity shops for books and resources to support your studies of the natural world.

Pond dipping is a really fun exercise to do with others and helps us to notice the detail. Do some research and organise an outing, being careful not to disturb the wildlife too much.

Make it more creative

Illustrate your writing.

Press flowers and leaves in your journal.

Glue some envelopes into your journal for gathering natural objects to use in other projects or just to keep.

Take it forward

When you get home, research what you have seen and try and answer your own questions, use the internet and your local community library,

Arrange a time to go back to the same place and notice any changes you notice.

The Royal Society for the Protection of Birds (RSPB) https://www.rspb.org.uk/ has information on identifying birds and wildlife, courses available, bird watching guides, bird identification guide and volunteering opportunities.

The Wildlife Trusts in the UK provide information on wildlife, wildlife gardening and run courses and events to help people connect with the natural environment https://www.wildlifetrusts.org/.

11. Haiku

This project involves writing about an experience in a short poem. At first I found it restricting and a bit frustrating, but with some practice I think it teaches us to be succinct and consider each word carefully.

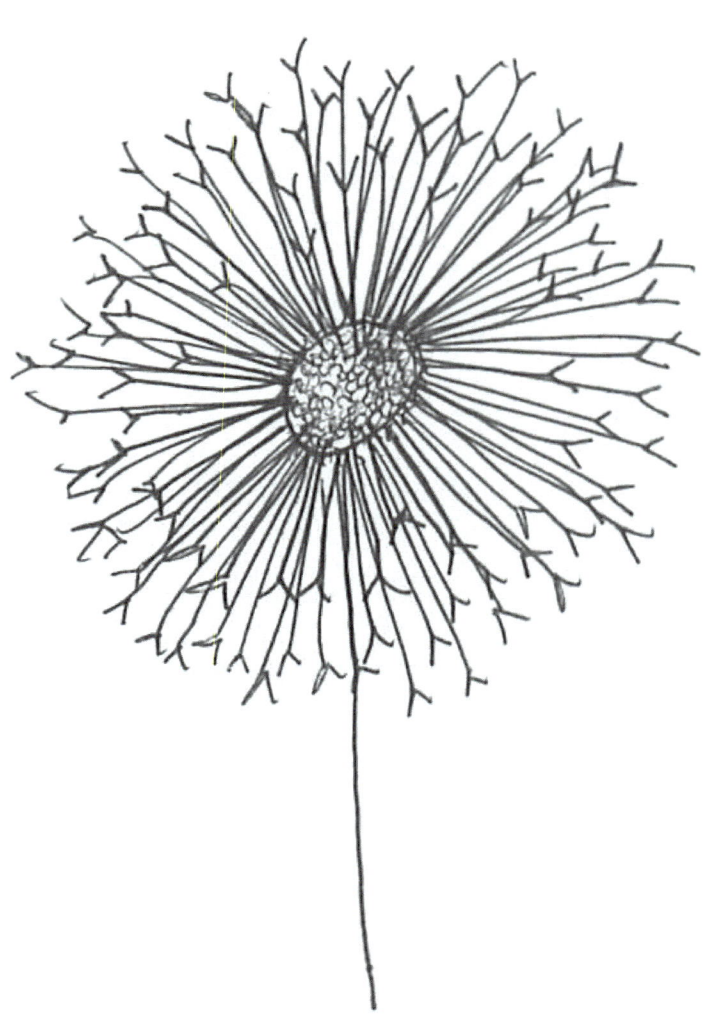

This project is mindful and connects us with nature, but there are suggestions for making it more social and creative below. The Haiku is a Japanese form of poetry that has 3 lines that do not rhyme and 15 syllables in the form of 5 in the first line, 7 in the second line and 5 in the last line. It can have a reference to nature or the seasons. It should leave the reader with a feeling or impression. It can have one verse or as many as you want. The Academy of American Poets (www.poets.org) describes the Haiku as "*Often focussing on images from nature, haiku emphasizes simplicity, intensity and directness of expression*" and there are lots of examples on this site. Below is my interpretation of the haiku poem with four verses and focussing on the seasons of the year.

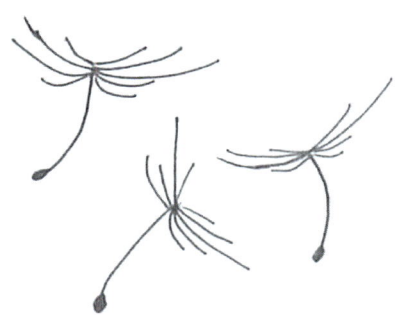

The seasons

First bright spring morning
The sun dances on water
I inhale warm joy

Late in summer's day
Cool river in between toes
Time flows by slowly

Grey autumn evening
The bonfire warms our fingers
Trees flame their leaves

Clear dark winter nights
Breath exhaled suspended
Green waits under snow

Jo Wren

Make it more social

Write a poem for someone that will be meaningful to them. This can be written in a card or just emailed or posted to let the person know you were thinking of them.

Make it more creative

Try different forms of poetry. Illustrate your poems. Write your poems on photographs you have taken of the moment. Embroider your poems onto textile pieces. Make a collage of pictures of your theme.

Take is forward

Visit www.thehaikufoundation.org or similar website to join or just read what others have written and the feedback.

Check Meetup to find a writing group near you.

III. Imagery writing

One of the ways of connecting more with nature that I've found useful is to take my journal out when I go for a walk somewhere beautiful in nature and take a moment to describe where I am in a short piece of writing that uses as many of the senses as possible. By doing this I find that I am naturally being more mindful as I am focussed on the present moment and not my thoughts.

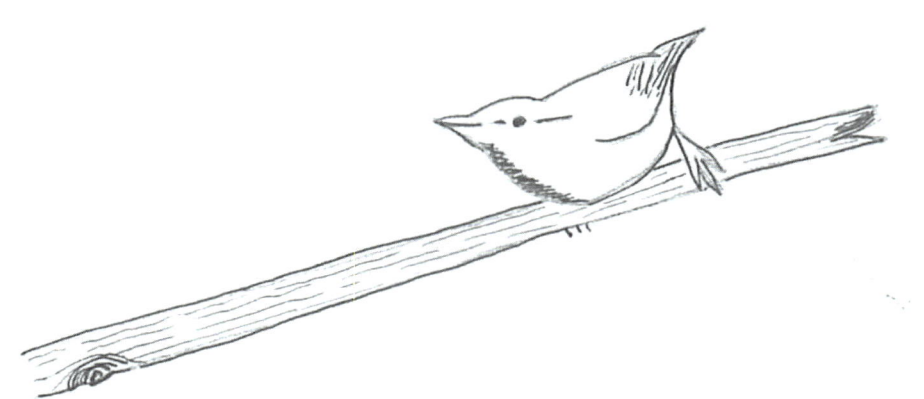

For this project go to a place of natural beauty with your journal and the aim is to be mindful in nature.

Take a few minutes to sit and connect with where you are and calm your breathing.

Describe in as much detail as possible what you are seeing, hearing, touching and smelling in a way that someone else might be able to imagine being there. Compare one thing with another to help you.

It doesn't have to be a long piece and I usually write in the third person but writing in the first person is also very effective. The use of adjectives and metaphors or similes where you are comparing one thing to another helps describe what you are experiencing and develop the right atmosphere. Thoughts and feelings evoked by what you are experiencing can help you to remember what it was like when you read back over your writing at a different time. This is a piece I wrote on a forest walk.

She sat resting on the soft, springy moss on a bank of earth deep in the forest. Her leg muscles warm and tingling from her walk. Under the canopy of leaves, the light was green tinted here, like looking through glass. Light pierced through the leaves forming a pool by her feet that rippled as the soft breeze made the trees shiver. She could smell the damp earth and slowly composting plants that hadn't survived through winter around her and was reminded of the predictable cycle of the seasons and life. From where she sat she could see a cluster of new primroses under a tree, their small cream flowers and vivid green leaves contrasting with the brown dead leaves the tree had shed the year before. They looked so delicate and fresh. She closed her eyes for a moment and listened to the sounds around her. She could hear the low whisper of the leaves above, the call of a nuthatch and the distant white noise hiss of a stream. She became aware of the sound of her breath calming as she rested. She felt like she was just where she should be at this moment. She enjoyed the peace a moment longer, and then moved on with her journey.

Jo Wren

Make it more social

Join or start a book club to explore literature you might not have chosen for yourself.

Join or start a writing group. Walk with other people and do the project together and discuss what you have written if you feel comfortable doing this.

Join an online writer's forum.

Make it more creative

Why not start with what you can see, hear, smell, touch and feel but then use your imagination to take the writing into a short fictional story.

Take photographs or illustrate your writing. Try writing within an illustration or shape of something relevant to your piece which might add another dimension to it.

Try different forms of writing.

Take it forward

There are lots of good examples of writing about the natural environment that you can look at for inspiration. I particularly like the descriptive language of Under Milkwood by Dylan Thomas and the opening chapter of Cider with Rosie by Laurie Lee, but explore for yourself pieces that evoke an image or series of images in your mind.

I really hope you have enjoyed either doing some of the projects in this resource or taking inspiration and going on your own journey. I hope you have managed to do more of the things that help you to feel and remain well. I would love to see some images of what you have created if you would like to share them, and any insights about what went well or how this resource could be improved. If you would like to share any images or comments, please Email me: jcwren@hotmail.co.uk or contact me via The Health and Well-being Initiative website with the contact form.

https://thehealthandwellbeinginitiative.wordpress.com

References

Cassou M and Cubley S (1995) Life, Paint and Passion. Reclaiming the magic of spontaneous expression. Jeremy P. Tarcher/Penguin, New York

Clark F, Azen S P, Zemk R, Jackson J, Calson, M, Mandel D, Hay J, Josephson K, Cherry B,Hessel C, Jocelynne P and Lipson L. (1997) Occupational Therapy for Independent-Living Older Adults: A Randomized Controlled Trial. *JAMA*, 278(16), pp1321-1326

College of Occupational Therapists. Recovering Ordinary Lives. The strategy for Occupational therapy in mental health services 2007-2017. A vision for the next ten years. Available at www.rcot.co.uk [Accessed 1st January 2019]

Cooper P (2018) Beats any drug that the doctors can give you. *Occupational Therapy News,* 26(8) pp16-17

Dynes R (1989) Using Creative Writing. *British Journal of Occupational Therapy.* 52(4)

Fearing VG, Law M, and Clark J (1997) An Occupational performance process model: Fostering client and therapist alliances. *Canadian Journal of Occupational Therapy,* 64 (1) p7-15

Finlay L and McKay E (2004) Mental illness:listening to users' experience. In L Findlay. *The Practice of psychological occupational therapy.* 3rd ed. Bath:Nelson Thornes

Genter, C, Roberts, A Richardson J and Sheaff M (2015) The contribution of allotment gardening to health and well-being: A systematic review of the literature. *British journal of Occupational Therapy*, 78 (10)

Gilbert P (2009) *The Compassionate Mind.* Constable, London.

Godfrey A (2000) Policy changes in the National Health Service: Implications and Opportunities for Occupational Therapists. *British Journal of Occupational therapy*, 63 (5)

Howard J. OT News (2017) Adding meaning to medicine. *Occupational Therapy News,* 25(6), pp22-24

Howard J (2018) further details about the service available at: https://www.yorkcvs.org.uk/ways-to-well-being/ [Accessed 12th December 2018]

Iwama M K (2006) *The Kawa Model: Culturally Relevant Occupational Therapy.* Elsevier, UK

Jon Kabat-Zinn (1979) Available at: https://www.mindful.org/tracking-the-skill-of-well-being/ [Accessed 10th October 2018]

Kielhofner G and Burke JP (1980) A model of human Occupation, Part 1. Conceptual framework and content. *American Journal of Occupational Therapy,* Sep;34(9): 572-81

Perruzza N and Kinsella EA (2010) Creative arts Occupations in therapeutic practice: a review of the literature. *British Journal of Occupational Therapy,* 73 (6)

Reilly M (1962) The Eleanor Clarke Slagle Lecture, *American Journal of Occupational Therapy,* XVI,1 pp. 1-9

Reynolds F (1997) Coping with Chronic Illness and Disability through Creative Needlecraft. *British Journal of Occupational Therapy,* 60(8)

Scriven A and Atwal A, (2004) Occupational therapists as Primary Health Promoters: Opportunities and Barriers. *British Journal of Occupational Therapist.* 67(10)

Wilcox AS (1998) *An Occupational perspective of health.* Thorofare, NJ:Slack

World Health Organisation (WHO) Mission statement. Available at:www.who.int/en/ [Accessed 6th January 2019)

World Health Organisation (2018) Mental Health: strengthening our response fact sheet. Available at: http://www.who.int/news-room/fact-sheets/detail/mental-health-strengthening-our-response [accessed 13th October 2018]

World Health Organisation (2012) Quality Rights tool kit: assessing and improving quality and human rights in mental health and social care facilities. Available at:http://www.who.int/mental_health/publications/QualityRights_toolkit/en/ [Accessed 1st September 2018]

Unruh AM, Smith N, and Scammell C(2000) The Occupation of gardening in life-threatening illness: A qualitative pilot study. *Canadian journal of Occupational Therapy,* 67(1)

5 Ways to Well-being. Available at: https://www.gov.uk/government/publications/five-ways-to-mental-well-being. [accessed 6th September 2018]

About the author

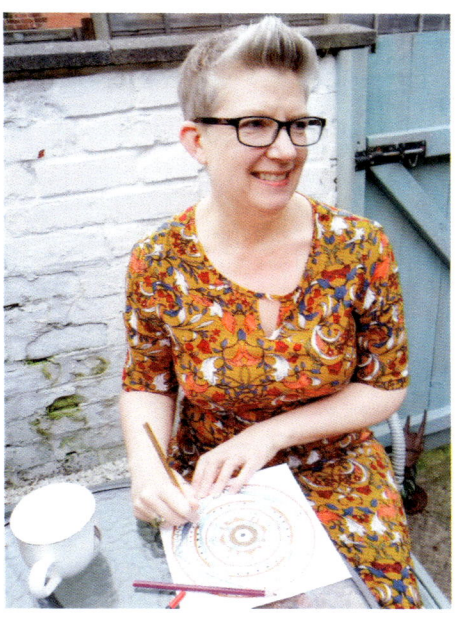

Jo is an experienced and passionate occupational therapist with a strong belief in the ability of others to achieve balance and success in their lives. She studied psychology at undergraduate level and health psychology at postgraduate level, worked in health research at the University of Manchester for several years, and qualified as an occupational therapist in 2007 after discovering the powerful role that occupational therapy plays in a person's well-being and recovery. Jo has experience working with people from a wide range of backgrounds, in different life circumstances and with different goals and aspirations. She is a strong believer in the importance of meaningful activity for good health and well-being and is the founding member of The Health and Well-being Initiative, an initiative led by four specialist occupational therapists in mental health aimed at anyone who wants to explore how to improve their health and well-being through meaningful activity. She is also Staff Health and Well-being Advisor for a mental health NHS Foundation Trust. Jo is a talented photographer and baker with a special interest in the role of nature in achieving well-being. She is a caring and compassionate person who enjoys working with people to support them to achieve their goals. She lives in Manchester with her dog Eric who graciously gave up his space on her lap during the writing of this resource.

Resources

Below is a list of sources of support in the United Kingdom. If you are outside the UK Befrienders Worldwide is a network of 400 international centres in 39 countries set up to help people who need emotional support to talk about problems in a confidential space.

Website: www.befrienders.org

Or find international help lines here

https://helplines.org/helplines/

If you are having suicidal thoughts and feel like acting upon them or have harmed yourself, this is a medical emergency so call 999 in the United Kingdom.

Call the NHS Helpline on 111 in the United Kingdom and staff will help you find the support and advice you need.

Age UK offers support for older people
Tel: 0800 055 6112 (England)
Tel: 0800 022 3444 (Wales)
Tel: 0800 124 4222 (Scotland)
Tel: 0808 808 7575 (Northern Ireland)

Alcoholics Anonymous is for anyone who is using alcohol excessively
Tel 0845 769 7555 (24 hours)
website: www.alcholics-anonymous.org.uk

Anxiety UK is a charity providing support if you've been diagnosed with an anxiety condition
Tel 03444 775 774 (Monday to Friday, 9.30am to 5.30pm)
Website: www.anxietyuk.org.uk

Aware is a helpline and email service for people experiencing depression in Northern Ireland
Tel: 028 9035 7820
Email: help@aware-ni.org

Beat offers support with eating disorders
Tel: 0808 801 0677 (adults)
or 0808 801 0711 (for under 18's)
website: www.b-eat.co.uk

British Association for Counselling and Psychotherapy (BACP) is a membership organisation that has an online directory of professional counsellors who will usually charge for their services
Website: www.bacp.co.uk

Bipolar UK is a charity helping people living with bipolar disorder or manic depression
Website: www.bipolarUK.org.uk

Campaign Against Living Miserable (CALM) a helpline specifically for men
Tel 0800 58 58 58 5pm to midnight every day

Carers UK offer support for unpaid carers
Tel: 0808 808 777 (England, Scotland and Wales)
or 028 9043 9843 (Northern Ireland)

Childline a helpline for children and young people under the age of 19
Tel 0800 1111

Cruse Bereavement Care offers support following a bereavement
Tel 0808 808 1677
website: www.crusebereavementcare.org.uk

Gamblers Anonymous offers support to people concerned about their own or someone else's level of gambling
Website: www.gamblersanonymous.org.uk

Living Life to the Full is a free online self help resource based on cognitive behavioural therapy
www.llttf.com

Mencap is a charity working with people with a learning disability, their families and carers
Tel: 0808 808 111 (Monday to Friday 9am to 5pm)
website: www.mencap.org.uk

The Mental Health Foundation provides information and support for anyone with mental health problems or learning disabilities
Website: www.mentalhealth.org.uk

Mind is a mental health charity that has information on conditions, resources and sources of support
Website: www.mind.org.uk

Narcotics Anonymous offers support to people who are concerned about their use of substances such as drugs
Tel: 0300 999 1212 (daily from 10am to midnight)
website: www.ukna.org

NSPCC is a children's charity dedicated to ending child abuse and child cruelty
Tel: 0800 1111 (24 hour helpline for children)
Tel 0808 800 5000 (24 hour helpline for adults concerned about a child)
website: www.nspcc.org.uk

No Panic is a charity offering support for people who have panic attack or obsessive compulsive disorder
Website: www.nopanic.org.uk

Refuge provide advice on dealing with domestic violence
Tel: 0808 2000 247 (24 hours)
website: www.refuge.org.uk

Relate is the United Kingdom's largest provider of relationship support
Website: www.relate.org.uk

Rethink Mental Illness offers support and advice for people living with mental illness
Website: www.rethink.org

The Royal College of Occupational therapist provides information on occupational therapy and a register of therapists
Website: www.rcot.co.uk

The Samaritans is a helpline for anyone who needs to talk
Tel: 116 123, Email: jo@samaritans.org
website: www.samaritans.org.uk

SAMH offers advice and support around mental health issues to anyone living in Scotland
Tel: 0141 530 1000 (9am-4.45pm)
Email: enquire@samh.org.uk

Sane offers emotional support, information and guidance for people affected by mental illness, their families and carers
Website: www.sane.org.uk/support

Silver Line is a helpline for older people
Tel 0800 4 70 80 90

Switchboard offers support and information around sexuality in the UK
Tel: 0300 330 0630
Email: chris@switchboard.lgbt

Veterans Gateway offers support for veterans/military personal and their families seeking support
Tel: 0808 802 1212, Text: 81212

Victim Support is for anyone in England and Wales affected by crime and provides confidential support and information, has an interpreter service for people who do not speak English and Next Generation Text for people who are deaf or hard of hearing 18001 08 08 16 89 111
Tel: 0808 16 89 111 (24 hours)

Printed in Great Britain
by Amazon

67101535R00072